# THE 49
# Professions of Joy

JACK KIRVEN

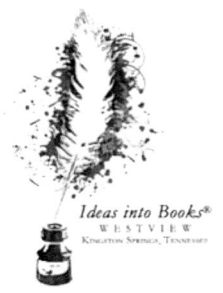

Copyright © 2020 Jack B. Kirven

All rights reserved, including the right to reproduction, storage, transmittal, or retrieval, in whole or in part in any form.

**Ideas into Books® WESTVIEW**
P.O. Box 605
Kingston Springs, TN 37082

www.publishedbywestview.com

ISBN 978-1-62880-208-5 Perfect Bound
ISBN 978-1-62880-202-3 Case Laminate
ISBN 978-1-62880-203-0 EBook

First edition, July 2020

Photo credits: Images used under license from Shutterstock.com.
The author gratefully acknowledges permission to reprint author photo: Bryan Bazemore, CPP.

Good faith efforts have been made to trace copyrights on materials included in this publication. If any copyrighted material has been included without permission and due acknowledgment, proper credit will be inserted in future printings after notice has been received.

Printed in the United States of America on acid free paper.

**Dedicated to:** Jennifer Hoff for unwavering and enthusiastic support for this expansive project.

**Thanks to**: Rose D., Sanna C., David K., Becky M., Valerie R., Rachel M., Helen M., Dean S., Jen W., Annie V., Jimmie C., Ron L., Dana J., Rob J., Kate S., Andrew C., Sibylle K., Dave P., Atticus T., Matt F., and Dan & Dave.

**Appreciation to**: All my beta readers and workshop guinea pigs — you improved this project. I dedicate Haiku #30 to all of you!

**Special Acknowledgement to**: RJB in Boston and MSS in Houston — your friendship, love, and encouragement make my life better. Thank you from my sincerest place of gratitude.

**Isabel** — I wish you could have seen this, because you would have loved it.

Engage further with this material:

- *Register to attend classes*
- *Book my workshops for your venue or event*
- *Receive discounts for group book orders*
- *Become certified in OM49: Learn to develop effective presentations*

Visit 49haiku.com
jack@INTEGRE8Twellness.com

The 49 Professions of Joy
@49Haiku
@49Haiku

Ebook design by Christina Snouwaert, Bluebird Design Agency, LLC.
bluebirddesignagency@gmail.com

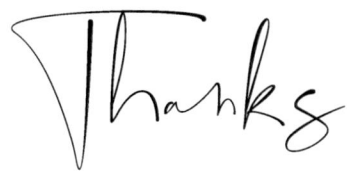

## You HAVE attended my immersive classes or workshops . . .

and I want to reiterate how much fun it was playing with you! I hope you experienced joy, spontaneity, curiosity, and insight. I encourage you to continue proactively engaging the chakras with all your senses, along with your mind. Remember to contemplate, practice, *and* enact!

I invite you to participate in the **Facebook Group**. Be sure to turn on your notifications! Here are some of the topics you'll find there:

- *We can share the poetry, prose, or stories we write.*
- *Let's ask questions and discuss empowering ideas.*
- *I'm sure many of us would enjoy describing activities we invent that purposefully align our chakras.*
- *Did you develop a new essential oil blend? We want to know the recipe!*
- *Have you found or created some music or art you think is inspiring? Show us!*
- *Any treats you like to eat? Definitely let us know about that: New sniffs and flavors are always exciting.*
- *I personally would love to know more about your practical experiences with gardening and homesteading.*

I hope this book will become your fond memento of our time together. It translates the multimodality of the class into a deeper exploration of the haiku, which zipped by so quickly in the soundscore! I talked about them at length, and this is an opportunity to let them shine. If you have any thoughts about them you want to share, I would love to know them. Please discuss them with me!

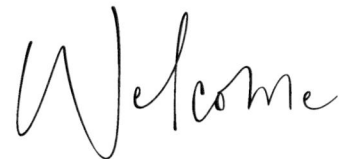

## You HAVE NOT attended my immersive classes or workshops . . .

but I want you to know how excited I am to share this pet project with you! Allow me to use this space to suggest how you might employ this book:

- *You do not need to read these pages in numerical order or in large chunks.*
- *Engage these concepts honestly — imagine how you could enact them. For example: Haiku #32 confronts gossip. What will you do to avoid, interrupt, or stop it in your home, school, group, or workplace?*
- *Read one color cycle at a time? Read one entry per day? Read only the haiku? Ignore everything except the one-sentence professions? Reread this content backwards? Open to any random page? Yes. Any method works.*
- *The colors, photos, poems, professions, anecdotes, explanations, and activities all point toward an entry's particular metaphor. This content is equally left-/right-brain.*
- *Some of what you experience as you contemplate yourself will be uncomfortable, and that is normal.*
- *This isn't only intellectual. Experience your senses. Translate the concepts into habits,*
- *experiments, or adventures.*
- *This is my own specialized matrix of chakras and Elementals. You will find different associations in different systems. They are all valid. Take what is helpful from each.*

I hope this book will become your companion as you take the journey of yourself. It does not have answers, and I am not a guru. You don't need anyone to tell you anything. You already know. Maybe this book can help you remember.

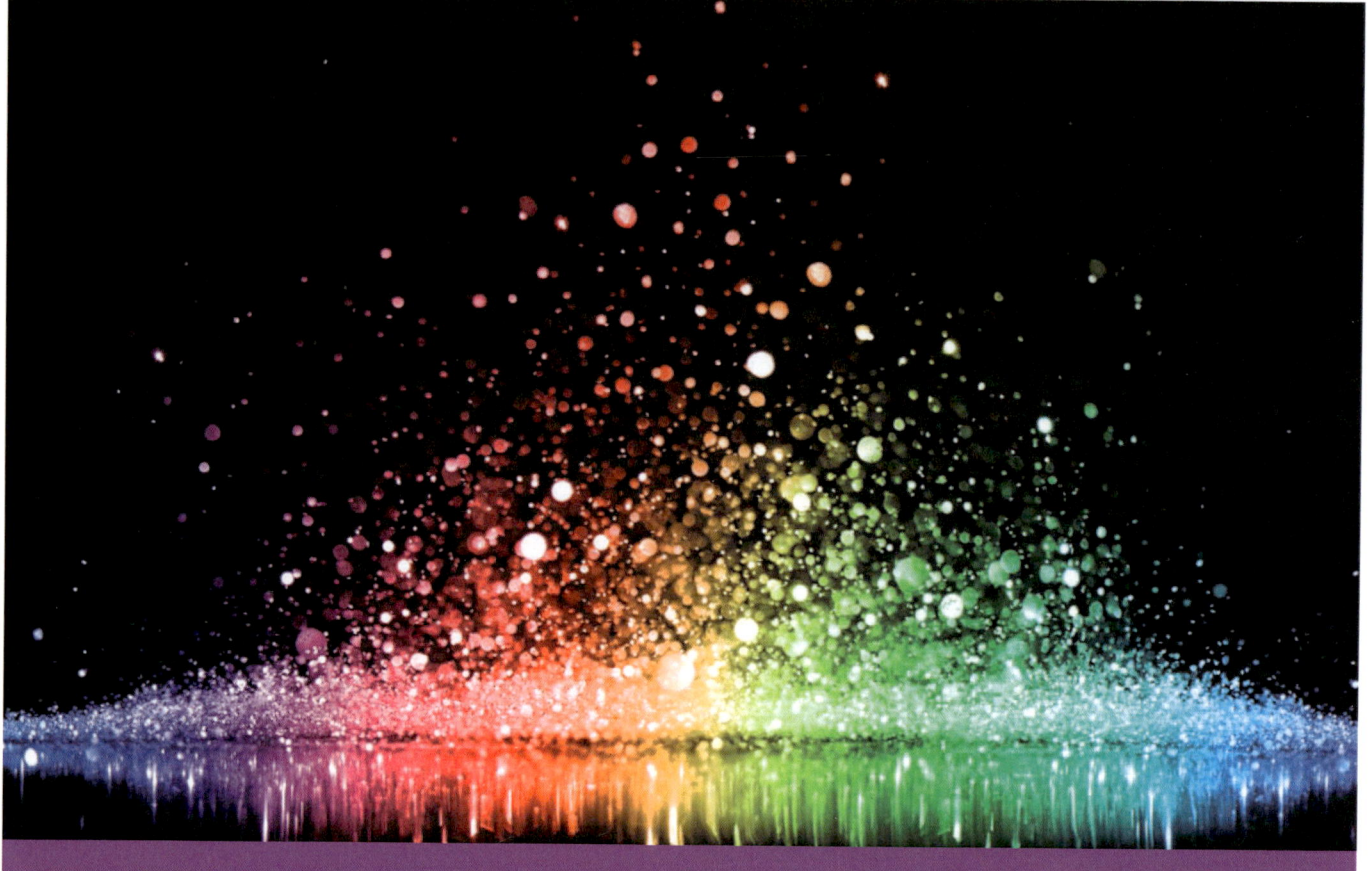

When you look at these beautiful colors, I have a question for you. Not which is your favorite. Not which one catches your eye. I want to know this: Which one are you drawn to most profoundly?

I'm purposefully asking you this now before I tell you in the subsequent sections what the colors signify. I don't want to "color" your perception of them — I'm middle aged, and I can tell Dad jokes in my own book, if I want to. If I were to say, "Red means this," you might be manipulated toward or away from it.

> **WHEN YOU LOOK AT THESE BEAUTIFUL COLORS, I WANT TO KNOW THIS:**
>
> Which one are you drawn to most profoundly?

Purposefully resist choosing the color that looks best to you based on your habitual preference. Which color do you feel compelled to return to repeatedly without hesitation? It could very well be your favorite, and that can have significance unto itself. But let your gut guide you more than your mind.

As your eyes drink, and without purposefully judging or pondering, simply pay attention to whether or not you notice any unexpected responses. If so, are they positive or negative reactions? Perhaps more than one color keeps beckoning to you? Right now I want you to home in on the one that has homed in on you.

Once you identify which color most insistently wants your attention, turn to the Table of Contents. Each chapter is associated with a color, as you will see from the chapter listing. Turn to that chapter, and see if the Professions in your color's cycle are relevant.

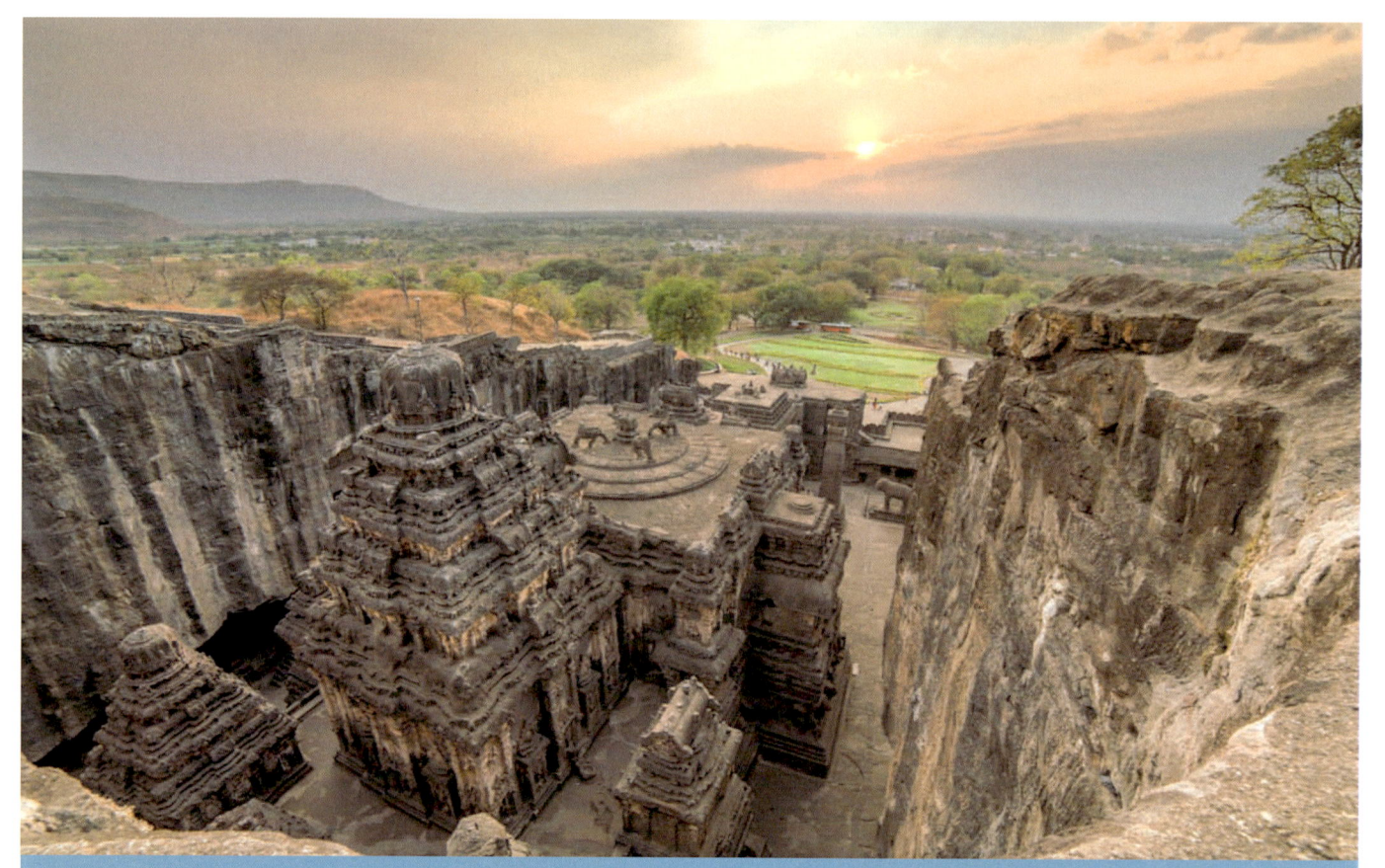

# TABLE OF
## *Contents*

| | |
|---|---|
| 10 | BACKSTORY |
| 12 | THE SEVEN ELEMENTALS |
| 14 | THE CHAKRAS |
| 14 | Muladhara |
| 30 | Svadisthana |
| 46 | Manipura |
| 62 | Anahata |
| 78 | Vishudha |
| 94 | Ajña |
| 110 | Sahasrara |
| 126 | ABOUT HAIKU |
| 128 | ADVICE FOR WRITING YOUR OWN |

# THE 49 PROFESSIONS OF JOY

## Backstory

This book represents a single layer of an immersive experience I designed, a group movement workshop for chakra alignment therapy. I began developing the class without realizing it in 1996. I began choreographing transitions between pictures of yoga asanas in order to create dance phrases. From 1997 to 2004 I studied crystal therapy, color therapy, light therapy, aromatherapy, drumming, haiku, and contact improvisation dance technique. In 2005 I bought (what at the time was) an exceedingly rare collection of seven quartz crystal singing bowls. I kept acquiring books, tools, and props, knowing they would all fit together somehow one day. Finally, I understood what I had been wanting to do: I spent all of 2019 and 2020 creating the aforementioned class.

Participants wanted to have ongoing access to the haiku from the soundscore. Although the poems seem "simple," they were not easy to write. Some blurted themselves in 15 minutes, others labored for 15 hours. I took entire weeks off from composing them at all, because the process is so exhausting. It took nine months to gestate all 49 haiku — it was like giving birth to a cube.

The first edition of this book was born during the global chaos of 2020. Talk about sudden bright lights, cold air, and a smack on the ass! I hope you embrace actionable serenity while you cradle this baby. My wish is for you to become a godparent to the proactive belief in mindful engagement throughout this potentially egalitarian world. We need people like you.

THE 49 PROFESSIONS OF JOY

# The Seven Elementals

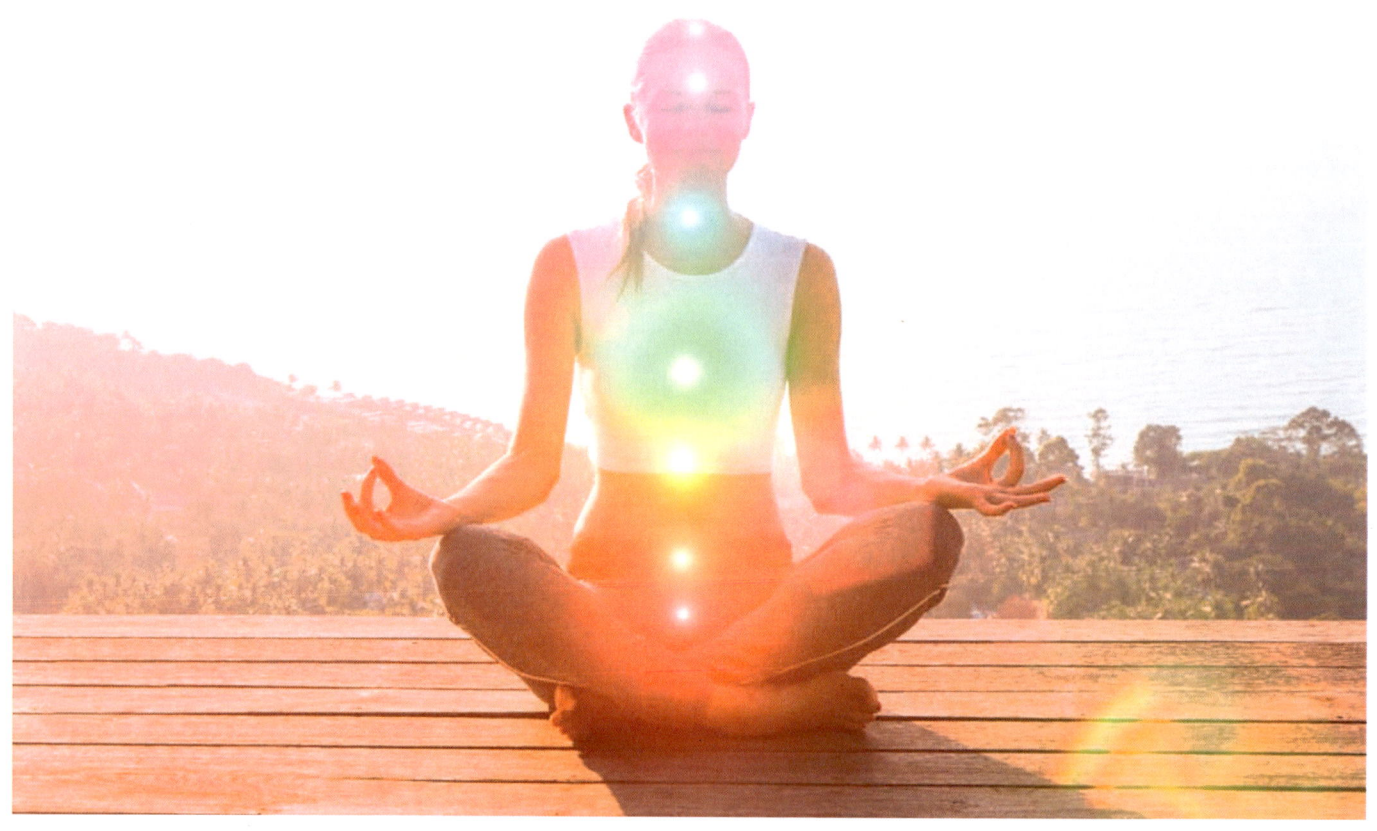

Elementals are a concept that seek to explain the nature and substance of reality. Qualities and characteristics of various materials become metaphors for everything within and beyond us. One familiar system is from Classical Greece, the ubiquitous Earth/Air/Fire/Water matrix. Different cultures have created various systems. The one in my class combines Western and Eastern influences, giving a system of seven Elementals (one for each chakra): Earth, Metal, Fire, Wood, Air, Water, and Akasha (the unity of All).

With this in mind, each chakra affects all the others. In this collection of poems, each cycle starts with the current chakra, then pairs its Elemental with those of all the others. There are seven haiku in each section. In this way I was looking for images that combine Elementals and then used that concept as a metaphor pertaining to a Profession of Joy. For example, Manipura (I DO) is related to that extraordinarily active Elemental, Fire. All the haiku in the Manipura collection will include concepts including fire, energy, or heat. Similarly, all those in Anahata (I LOVE) are connected to plants, because the Elemental for the heart chakra is Wood.

To illustrate the example of this particular combination, Profession #16 of 49 uses forest fires as an example of how Fire (I DO) touches Wood (I LOVE): *"I profess that — I DO — appropriate reckonings of my relationships."*

## SCORCHED DEVASTATION:
## RAVAGED FORESTS KINDLE GROWTH.
## FECUND, OPEN, KEEN.

*Although temporarily disruptive, exiting dead end relationships ushers productive connections.*

**COLOR**
RED

**ELEMENTAL**
EARTH

**PURPOSE**
GROUNDING

**MANTRA**
"I AM"

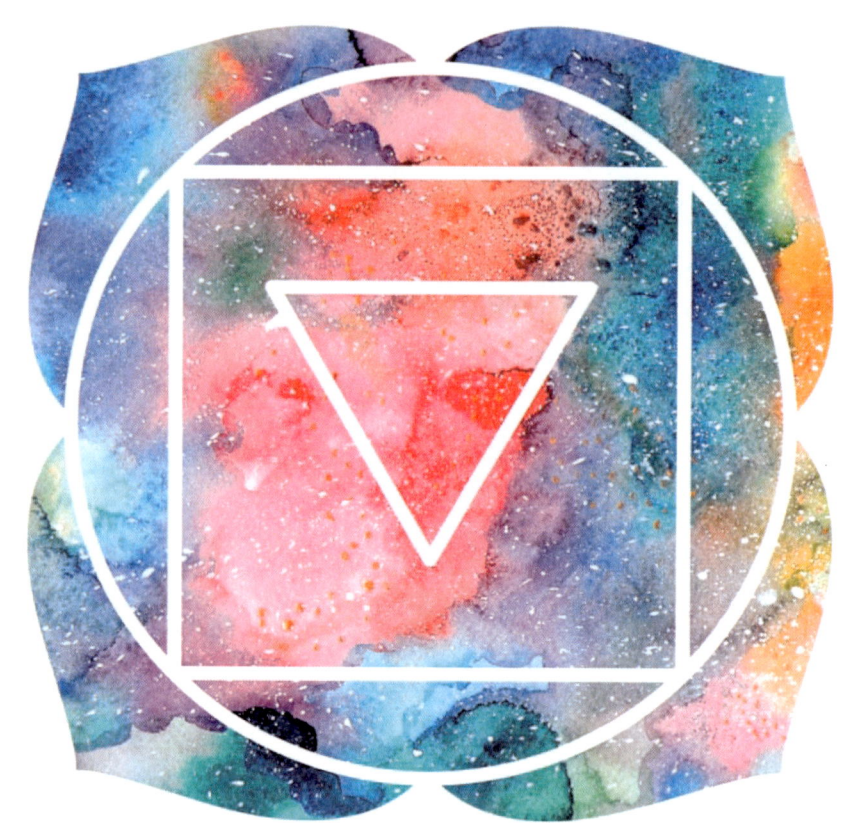

MULADHARA
*Intro*

Also called the Root Chakra, this energy vortex is located at your pelvic floor. When you sit down, directly beneath you is where this powerful wheel creates your overall balance. When it is healthy and aligned you will enjoy a strong column supporting all the rest. Health, safety, stability, and plenty rest on this solid foundation.

When it is misaligned your perception of well-being is undermined. Illness, fear, chaos, and poverty mentality seep from a cracked bedrock. But is there too much energy crumbling it, or not enough energy allowing it to sink and fracture?

The first cycle of *The 49 Professions of Joy* redefines how you create your reality. According to Maslow's Hierarchy of Needs, until you feel healthy and safe, you cannot prioritize anything else. This is your opportunity to provide fundamentals for yourself, especially if you feel you cannot trust anyone else to help you. In fact, you should generate that internal resilience yourself. It can then be nourished by your external relationships. First get right with your internal relationship. Balance exercise with innercise!

A practice that has helped me is writing with specificity, literally defining my intentions. It gives me a target for my energy, drawing my focus away from fear. I am not asking you to put your faith in any particular concept of direct and immediate attraction. What I am encouraging you to remember is that where you put your attention is where you put your action. Proactively envision your unique, ideal life.

Stars? Dust. Salt, earth, clay.

Me? Life's vase birthing diamonds.

Clay? Earth. Salt, dust, stars!

# #1 OF 49

## I PROFESS THAT — I AM — THE STUFF OF ETERNITY.

### MULADHARA: EARTH (I AM) TOUCHES MULADHARA: EARTH (I AM)

Material combinations create your entire self. Your constituent parts come from the building blocks of the universe, which stars generate during their own lives. Ultimately you return to that universal stuff. It's romantic to say we come from star dust. It's truly a beautiful way to understand your connection to the world and creation.

Even your thoughts and memories exist in the physical world. Experiences trigger chemical reactions that fire and wire your neurons. These impressions change the shape of surface proteins in your brain. They are encoded into the microscopic physical bodies that make up your mind. Memories are tangible records, so thoughts literally become things.

So why not process all the pressures and stresses constructing your memories as an opportunity to produce wise gemstones? You are made of carbon. Diamonds are, too. Why not make the metaphorical leap and understand that you physically build your life with the thoughts you think? You are as tough as stone. Build your being with diamonds.

*Related entries: Haiku #15 & Haiku #44*

Instinct, pleasure, joy:

Chiseled inside my body's

firm, sculptured delight.

# #2 OF 49

## I PROFESS THAT — I AM — A MONUMENT TO SENSUALITY AND HAPPINESS.

### MULADHARA: EARTH (I AM) TOUCHES SVADISTHANA: METAL (I FEEL)

You are a physical manifestation of response and memory. What created them? Your senses. Your injuries. Your recoveries. Your emotions. The physical form your true self wears like fleshy armor is the conduit funneling your experience into your perception. And although our senses are woefully limited, they are also marvelously nuanced.

Invest and enrich yourself with as much detail as you can. What are the notes in that chord? What scents are mixing together to create that aroma? Do you feel you can trust this person? Why are you anxious? Walk backwards through the steps until you know the moment your bell rang. Of all the myriad ways to touch or be touched, which do you crave most?

That word "firm" in the haiku obviously has a sexual connotation. However, beyond firm butts, muscles, nipples, and fiddly bits, you yourself must be firm. Stay strong. Be constant. Remain yourself. And yet, when can a better version of you be chiseled out from the rocky chaff? Become the wondrous, revealed masterpiece.

*Related entry: Haiku #14*

Cerebral kiln, burn!

Mix mortar! Seize your trowel!

Mason, set your bricks!

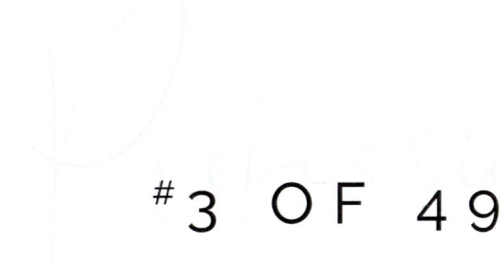

# #3 OF 49

## I PROFESS THAT — I AM — THE ARCHITECT WHO BUILDS MY LIFE.

**MULADHARA: EARTH (I AM)** TOUCHES **MANIPURA: FIRE (I DO)**

You are what you think. You are what you feel. And you are what you do. Your actions propel you into the cycle of cause and effect. Deeds construct your legacy.

Does telling people who you are suffice? You generally have to show them. You do that by first defining for yourself who you want to be. How will you transform yourself into this person? What do you have to accomplish to make it so?

Notice that the word "set" in the haiku isn't only a call to action. It isn't a bland imperative to put something into place, but to perform energetically with ambitious resolve. Obviously we can become too set in our ways, but first we have to have ways! Right?

Those purposeful exclamation points: Reread that with periods instead. Where is the energy? Without enthusiasm your work will be dull. Do you live an exclamation point life? Are you using your agency confidently? Is your work empowering and enriching you? Your answer reveals your truth.

*Related entry: Haiku #21*

Claim YOUR hewn temple.

Hand carved, blessed living marble:

Call MY heart YOUR home.

# #4 OF 49

## I PROFESS THAT — I AM — A COMPASSIONATE, SACRED SPACE.

### MULADHARA: EARTH (I AM) *TOUCHES ANAHATA: WOOD (I LOVE)*

When Earth meets Wood, you can build a dwelling. Or a shrine. But also consider that broken or damaged hearts can seem stoney. The point here is that when you successfully carve out Anahata's temple within yourself, you manifest a sacred space. You honor your own spirit in opening it to others. You share your best gift: Yourself.

When you invite someone in, whether it be for romantic love or any type of trusting relationship, you have invited them to enter what is effectively a home for the gods. Namaste: The divine in Me recognizes the divine in You, and I am trusting You to reciprocate. Let Us honor Our Selves.

Home is your sancta sanctorum. Hopefully it is the place where you can be unequivocally you. Here you are at your most secure, but also your most vulnerable. Not only literally, but metaphorically as well. Who are you going to allow to amble through while you lounge in your spiritual underwear? Home is where the heart is.

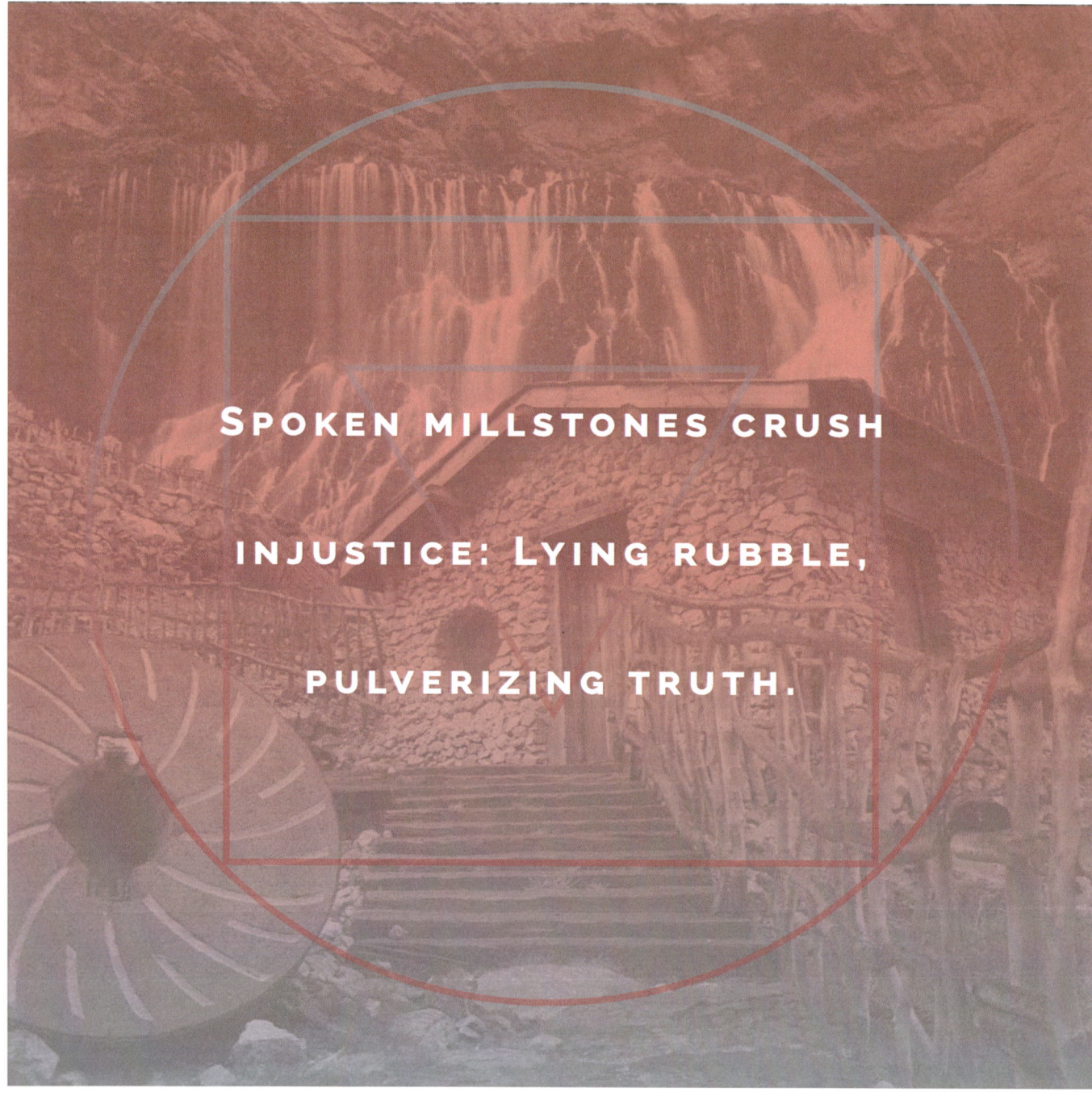

# #5 OF 49

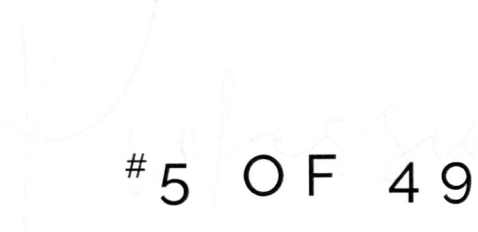

## I PROFESS THAT — I AM — THE WORDS THAT RING TRUE.

**MULADHARA: EARTH (I AM)** *TOUCHES* **VISHUDHA: AIR (I SAY)**

The mantra for the fifth chakra, Vishudha, is I SAY. This isn't limited to spoken words. Clear expression includes any creative projects or impulses that come from a place that communicates the authentic self's honest intent.

When your Root Chakra is balanced and you are secure in yourself, you are able to speak truth to power. This does not imply that marginalized or disempowered people cannot be honest or outspoken. Far from it. But if you do enjoy privilege of whatever kind, it should be your duty to use your voice to advocate for equality. If those whose circumstances are more humble than your own can do it, you certainly can.

"Lying" is the word of note here. The rubble is scattered or strewn about, but it also exudes lies, which are a manifestation of an imbalance in Vishudha. Lying versus standing. Lying versus truth telling. Lies are laid waste. In case it helps clarify the metaphorical connection between Earth and Air, pulvis is Latin for dust. Even gentle breezes immediately scatter motes.

Sowing clarity:

Seeds sprout, shoots thrive, truth blossoms.

Wisdom reaps sage fruit.

# #6 OF 49

## I PROFESS THAT — I AM — VISION'S FERTILE GARDEN.

### MULADHARA: EARTH (I AM) TOUCHES AJÑA: WATER (I SEE)

The obvious metaphor for Earth touching Water is gardens. I would point out that Ajña is located at your Third Eye, at the center of your brow. The seeing here isn't in the literal sense. Do you see what I'm saying? This is the function of Ajña, so this particular garden isn't cultivating relationships — that comes up in *Haiku #28* — but rather cultivating ideas, harvesting broad learning, and seeing the world as it is.

I would like to point out the word play for "sage." It is a synonym for wise. Learning happens only when your immediate needs are met. When you don't have to worry yourself about safety or survival, you can put your resources toward the mental, as opposed to having to preoccupy yourself with the physical. Muladhara has to be stable for Ajña's eye to open. Also, sage is a plant that grows out of rich soil, and it can be gathered into bundles. These sage smudge sticks are used to smoke bad juju out of enclosed places.

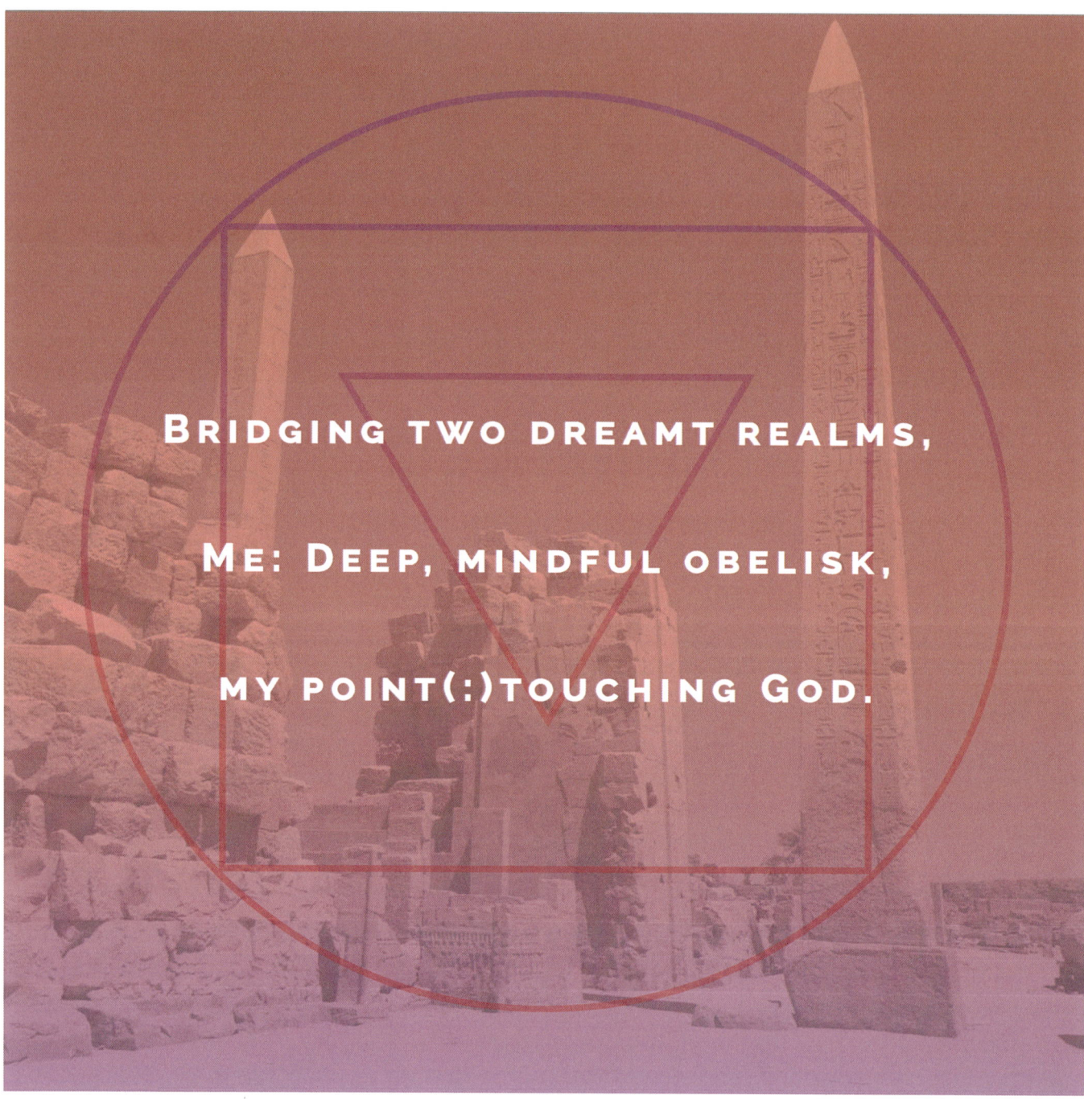

# #7 OF 49

## I PROFESS THAT — I AM — A CONNECTION BETWEEN HEAVEN AND EARTH.

### MULADHARA: EARTH (I AM) *TOUCHES* SAHASRARA: AKASHA (I KNOW)

Akasha, meaning æther, symbolizes the most spiritual quality of the chakras. You need not adhere to any religion to align Sahasrara. You need only value understanding your reason for being here, and defining the moral code that extends your spirit out into the world around you.

We ourselves bridge profane and divine. We conceive and inhabit both realms. We remember those who pass before us, saying they enliven memories. We give them continued existence. But do they not also remember us? Do they not also give us existence? Why be concerned with preserving legacies otherwise? We are obelisks, standing firmly here, reaching contemplatively there.

I avoided "grounded" and "rooted" in favor of "deep" and "mindful" as synonyms with far more nuance: Deep core, deep thought, mindful acts, mindful meditation, etc. Flesh and spirit combine.

That creative punctuation: Let me explain. The (:) gives the option of pausing. It changes the literal (earthly) to the conceptual (spiritual). No spaces before or after (:) bridges both readings simultaneously, uniting base to point.

*Related entry:* **Haiku #44**

**COLOR**
ORANGE

**ELEMENTAL**
METAL

**PURPOSE**
SENSING

**MANTRA**
"I FEEL"

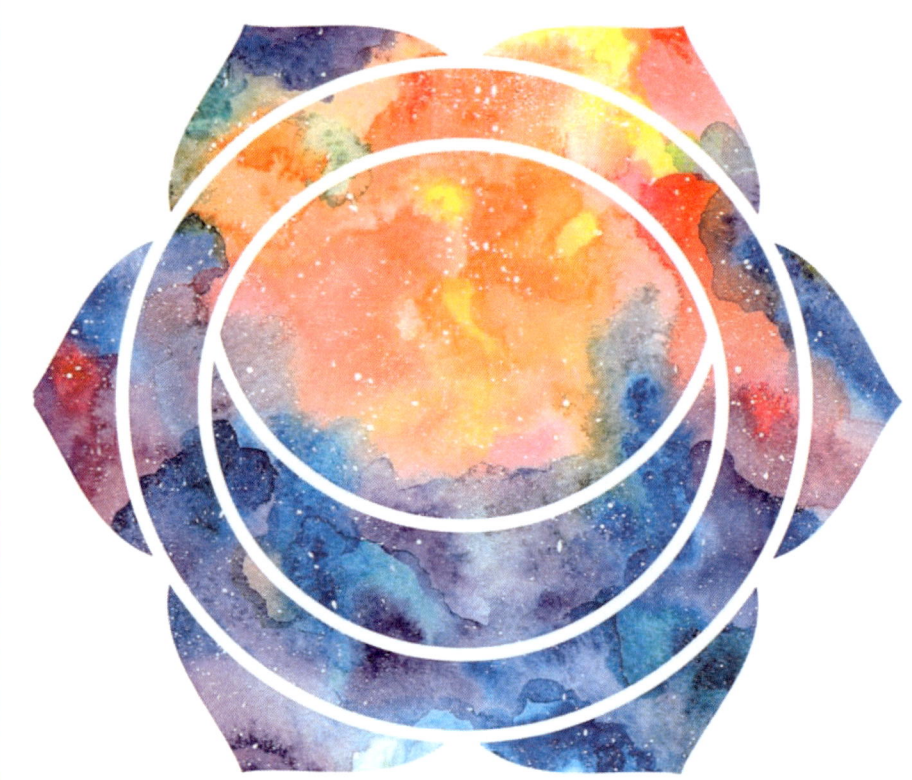

SVADISTHANA
*Intro*

Also called the Sacral Chakra, this energy vortex is located between your pubic area and bellybutton. You have probably heard the phrase, "I just feel it in my gut." That is where the intuitive concept "feels" appropriate, yes? When it is healthy and aligned you will trust and accept your senses. Various pleasures, like sensuality or sensorial enrichment, instinct, and fulfillment reside in your viscera.

When it is misaligned your perception of happiness is undermined. Various pains, numbness, shame, guilt, doubt, and hunger gurgle in an irritable bowel. But is there too much energy bloating it, or not enough energy starving it?

The second cycle of *The 49 Professions of Joy* redefines how you relish your physical, emotional, and spiritual bodies. I want you to think beyond sex and romance here. Those are essential components of a healthy life; however, I am asking you to enjoy in proper measure the pleasures you indulge. Beyond physical senses, listen to your instinct. Release taboos that serve any unhelpful purpose, while maintaining your sense of decency, kindness, and fairness.

It is common to learn shame about sex, physical appearance, and confidence. Explore your body by yourself. Explore it with others, encouraging everyone involved to feel physical and emotional bliss. Be honest about what you can and cannot "improve" in your physical appearance: Grow where you can, accept where you cannot. Also recognize the difference between pride and arrogance: Pride is self love based on truth, and arrogance is self love based on fear.

WHETTED: MY KEEN BLADES SHRED DULL ILLUSIONS, SLICING OBTUSE DECEPTIONS.

# #8 OF 49

## I PROFESS THAT — I FEEL — MY TRUSTWORTHY INTUITION GUIDING ME.

*SVADISTHANA: METAL (I FEEL) TOUCHES SVADISTHANA: METAL (I FEEL)*

Svadisthana is feeling in all its rawest forms, including emotions. All your five senses and their perceptions are here.

Your sixth sense is intuition. It remains as vital to your survival and happiness as any of the others. I feel comfortable. I feel I should leave. I feel you lie to me. I feel this option is right.

When you ponder, answers come instantaneously. Should I do this? NO! Is this wise? YES! Everything afterward cuts toward apologetics, justification, excuses, or doubt.

Can our senses deceive us? Definitely, yes. But trouble comes when we refuse to consider our inner voices. Often when I ignored my gut, I experienced terrible predicaments. Situations I would never wish on anyone. I frequently brushed aside first impressions, because I feared being rude or judgmental, only to find myself needlessly endangered. I am not saying you should invest in mistrust, paranoia, or bigotry. I am telling you to pay attention. If something alarms you, are there valid reasons? Appreciate the distinction between being prejudiced versus judicious.

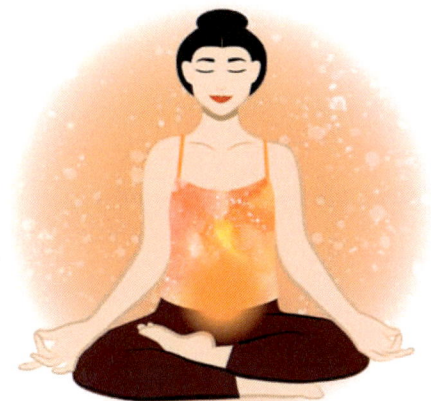

*Related entry: Haiku #16*

Apt iron, rapt zeal:

Preparing. Opulent meal,

savoring. Ordeal?

# #9 OF 49

## I PROFESS THAT — I FEEL — RESPONSIBILITY IS MY FIRST CHOICE.

### SVADISTHANA: METAL (I FEEL) TOUCHES MANIPURA: FIRE (I DO)

When Metal contacts Fire, cooking renders both useful. By allowing our emotions and instincts to contain and direct our choices, we give ourselves a way to act meaningfully, productively. This metaphor examines feeling as context for doing.

Too often our emotions boil over, and we make unsavory choices. When do you need to turn up the heat to do more, and when should you simmer to do less? Your feelings affect your actions by way of interrupting them to first consider empathy and consequence.

Patiently preheat the pan. Build a little heat. You are not cooking yet. You prepare to act. Anticipate the recipe's every step, every consequence. If you understand the ingredients and any substitutions, you will be able to respond to all sorts of situations. You can predict and avoid many problems. What ordeal? Where?

Would you eat this meal? If not, why make it? Are you willing to own what you are about to do? If you hesitate taking responsibility for the action, should you even be doing it?

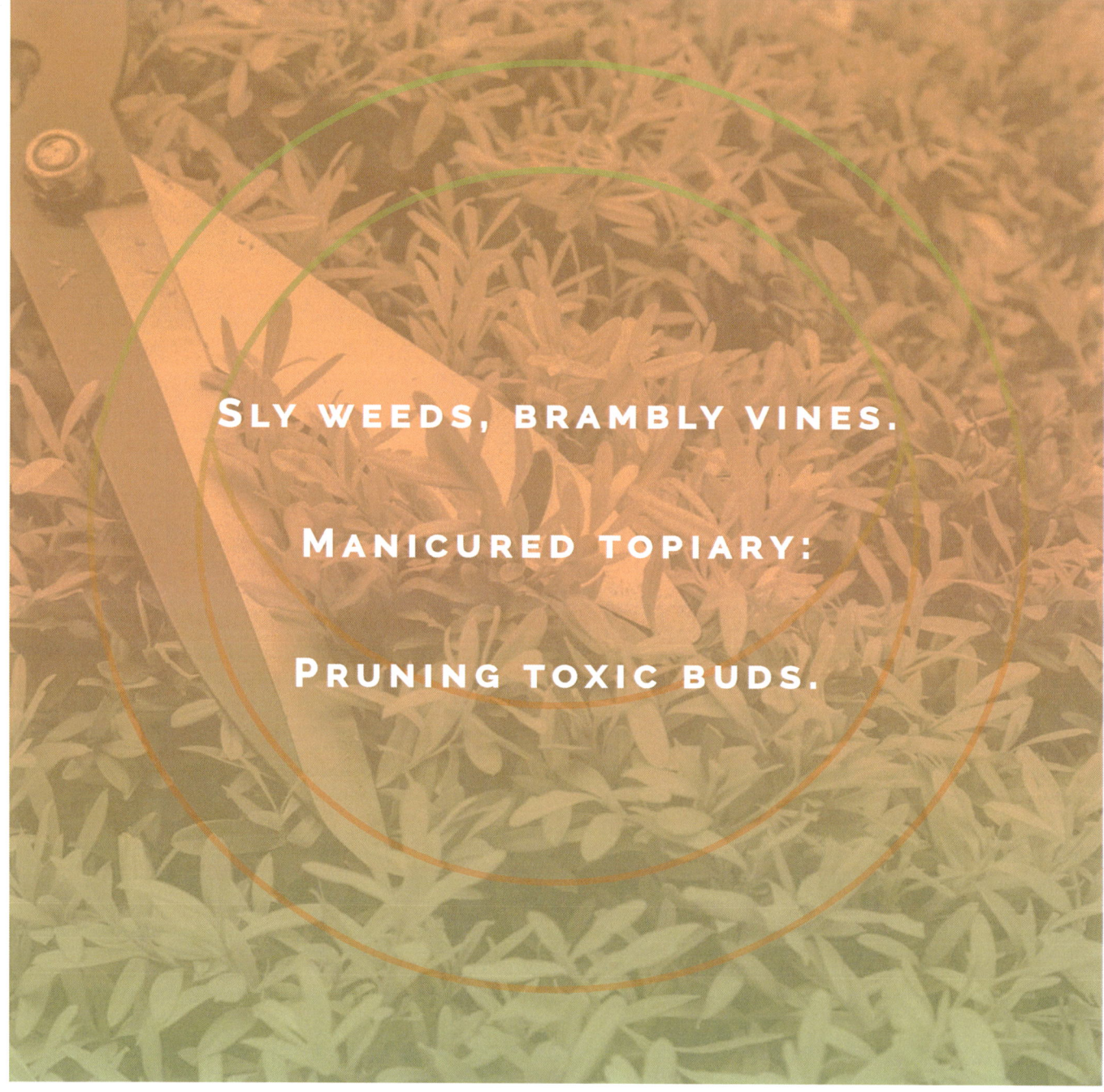

# #10 OF 49

## I PROFESS THAT — I FEEL — THAT ONLY THE DESERVING DESERVE MY LOVE.

*SVADISTHANA: METAL (I FEEL)* TOUCHES *ANAHATA: WOOD (I LOVE)*

Let's be very honest: Most people have far too many "friends." Very often these "friends" are totally superfluous at best and destructive at worst. You can comfortably know only around 150 people at any moment. This is Dunbar's Number. Of those 150, you fill roughly 67% of your heart space bonding with only 15. Of the maximum number of people with whom you can sustain a healthy social relationship, only 10% are your friends.

Amercian English is particularly unhelpful in this regard. We abuse the word friend to a degree that makes me cringe. Frequently, someone I just met (who isn't even sure of my name) will introduce me to others as their friend.

Be picky. Understand the term "friend" as the French do. You might have many pleasant acquaintances (connaissances) and several good buddies (copains), but only a very select few friends (amis). Avoid abusing the word friend. When you call a person a friend, let that, in and of itself, be the best compliment you could give them.

*Related entries: Haiku #16 and Haiku #21*

Dulcet, silver flute:

Exhale… trill fair melodies.

Hush life's verbose gales.

# #11 OF 49

## I PROFESS THAT — I FEEL — THAT MY EXPRESSION OF MYSELF IS POWERFUL.

*SVADISTHANA: METAL (I FEEL)* TOUCHES *VISHUDHA: AIR (I SAY)*

Despite being a former flautist, when I came to this combination of Elementals, the first image I considered was wind chimes. But in my mind that puts the source of communication out into the world, and then comments on the way in which the words of others move our emotions. I wanted to consider the emotive wind propelled out of one's self.

Sharing your feelings is a crucial part of maintaining emotional alignment. Whether it be with singing, speaking, writing, dancing, art, therapy, or any other expressive pursuit, giving your insides a breath of fresh air keeps them healthy and flowing. But what do you say, and how do you say it?

Your "voice" can be a source of peaceful breezes or terrifying blasts. Either way, what you express is powerful. Your words matter. They affect the world, so use them appropriately. No, the melody isn't always a warbling birdsong. Sometimes you do need to blast a shrill whistle. Be especially mindful of songs you play about yourself.

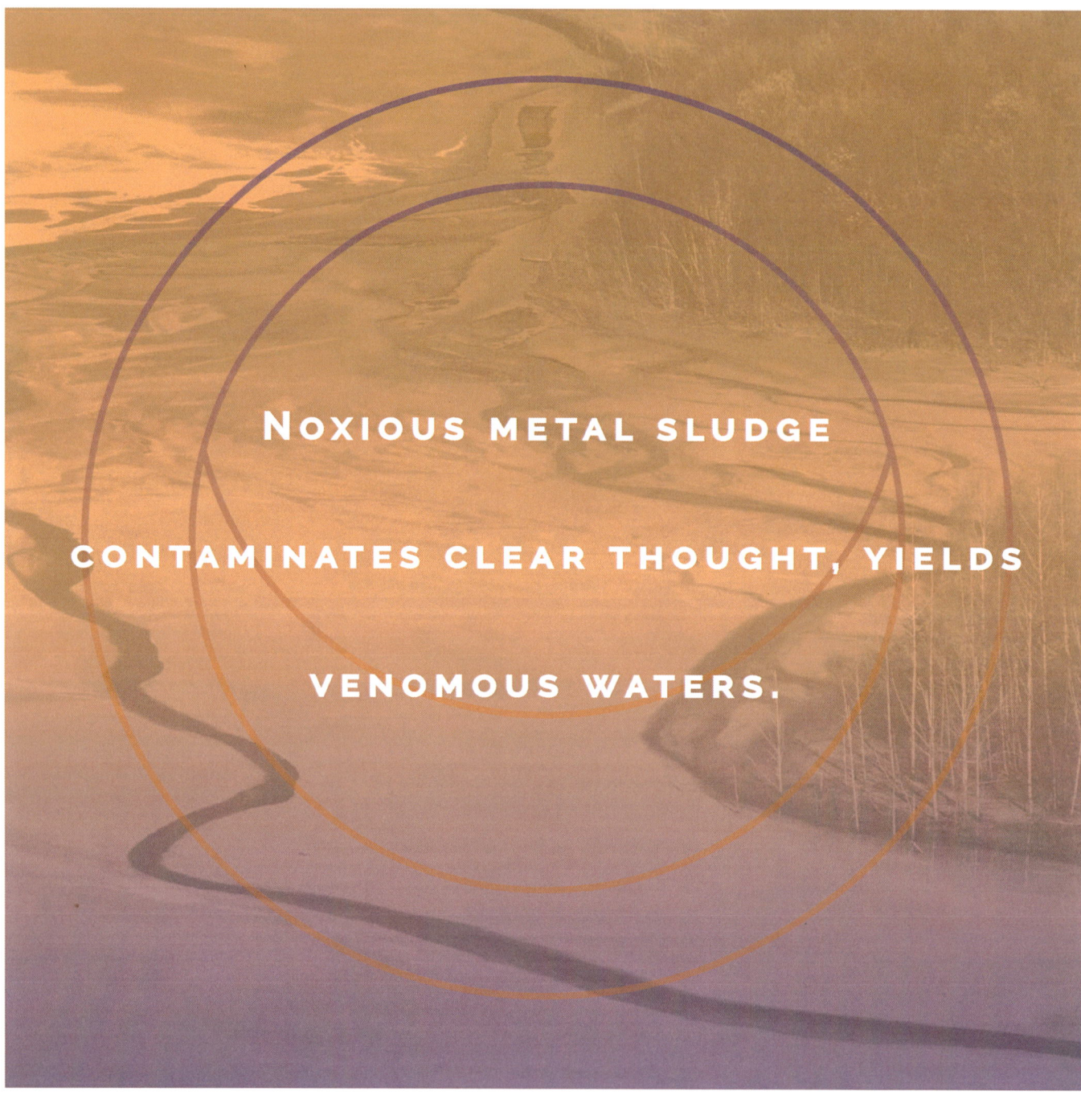

# #12 OF 49

## I PROFESS THAT — I FEEL — NO OBLIGATION TO DRINK THE POISONOUS THOUGHTS OF OTHERS.

*SVADISTHANA: METAL (I FEEL)* TOUCHES *AJÑA: WATER (I SEE)*

These are strange times, no point looking past it. I would posit that much of the mercurial poison polluting the world's political currents has been dumped there by toxic feelings like fear, bigotry, and greed. These then contaminate the way we think about and see each other. Don't drink the Kool-Aid, man!

Now that I write this, I wonder why I did not think to use blood as the metaphor. A fluid full of iron that symbolizes both health and violence? It would have been perfect.

Coming back around to thinking about conflict as pollution, what can be done to restore our streams? How do we clean our streams of thought? How do we filter out the heavy metals spewing like sewage from the bowels of nationalist thought?

It's hard to hate a group once you more intimately know someone from that group. My suggestion: Literally, share some drinks with someone unlike yourself and talk with them. Learn to understand them and how they see the world.

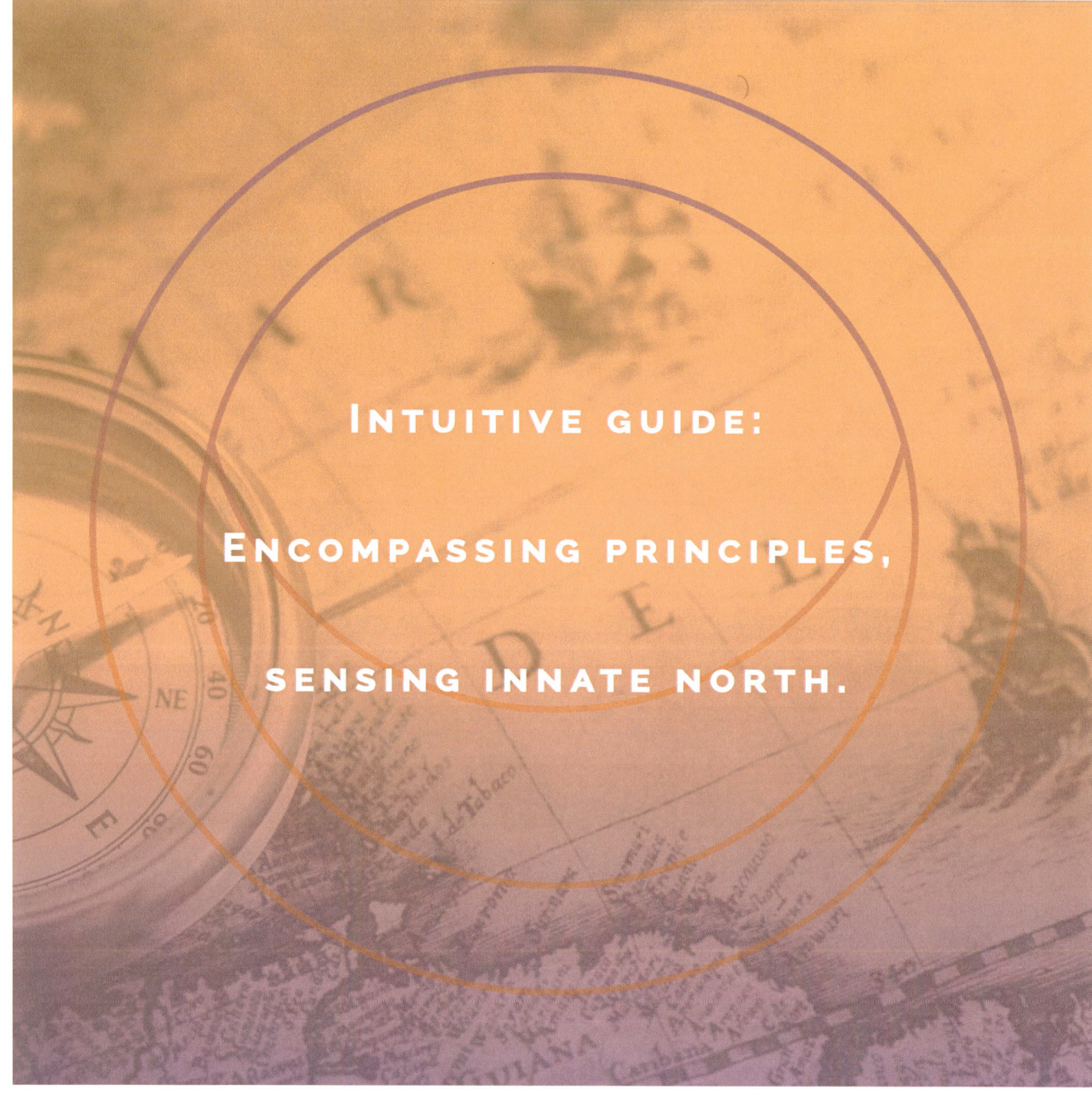

# #13 OF 49

## I PROFESS THAT — I FEEL — MY MORAL CODE AIMING ME CORRECTLY.

**SVADISTHANA: METAL (I FEEL)** TOUCHES **SAHASRARA: AKASHA (I KNOW)**

See what I did there with encompassing? Of course you did, clever traveler! When you encounter the individual haiku that include Sahasrara, and especially the Sahasrara cycle itself, the Elementals take on a more spiritual quality. And what is the spiritual equivalent of feeling? It is morality.

Beyond the instinct of self preservation, intuition guides us from one experience to the next as we navigate relationships and situations. Why does a civilization continue? Because people agree to follow its direction. Ultimately all our explorations are possible only because we decide we value stability more than chaos. For successful coexistence, cultures define basic precepts concerning autonomy, respect, and justice.

There are bad actors, obviously. But there are so many more good actors. I firmly believe that people are doing their best. For some people that is not very good; however, I choose to accept people as generally well intended. I know you want to do your part, and that is why I believe you do what is right as much as you possibly can.

Lewd! You exude, ooze.

Adored golden mother lode,

snugly engulfed plug.

# #14 OF 49

## I PROFESS THAT — I FEEL — PLEASURE WITHOUT SHAME.

### SVADISTHANA: METAL (I FEEL) TOUCHES MULADHARA: EARTH (I AM)

I often direct people beyond sex. I repeatedly assert that sensuality exceeds sexuality. This is not prurience. It is respecting the economy of language and space I allowed myself. I cannot dedicate full chapters to each feeling, so all are necessarily blended. I feel gratified by structured discipline. However…

If this haiku makes you squirm for any reason, I achieved my goal: Feel something! Let us just rut about in lustful abandon for a moment. Sex is extraordinarily and unnecessarily complicated. Simplify it.

The poem's vowels are pornographic by design. You just went back to read only the vowels, didn't you? Did you find you had to do it quietly? I am giggling remorselessly at your blushes.

Your body is a matrix of nerves existing only for stimulation. In and of themselves they have no morality. We are the ones getting in the way of our fulfilled, sated gratification. In **Haiku #2** of 49, you were the monument sculpted by pleasure. In #14, you are the delight moving through your own body.

**COLOR**
YELLOW

**ELEMENTAL**
FIRE

**PURPOSE**
EMPOWERING

**MANTRA**
"I DO"

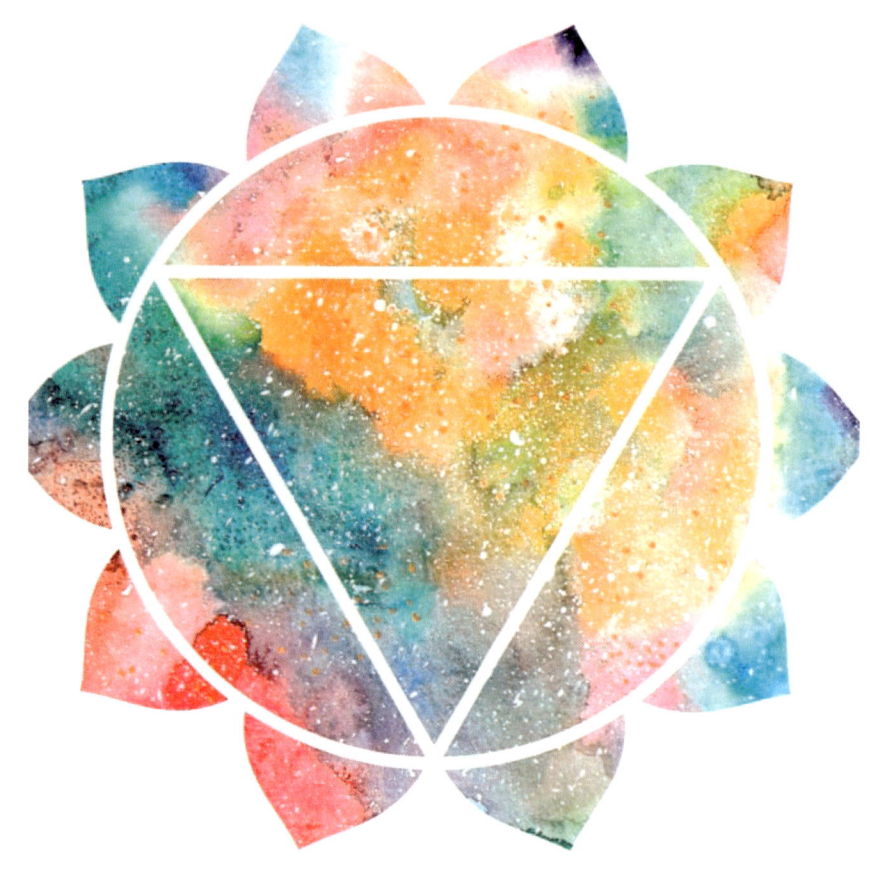

# MANIPURA

Also called the Solar Plexus, this energy vortex is located between your bellybutton and heart. You have probably heard the phrase, "I have a fire in my belly." It means you are eager to do something, and that is appropriate. All action begins in your center. Before you can make any movement, you must first activate and stabilize your core (your "belly," as it were). When it is healthy and aligned you will have momentum. Purpose, ambition, concentration, and focus are burning in your stomach — you feed the flame of action with intention.

When it is misaligned your embers burn low with apathy, lethargy, distraction, and self-imposed obstacles. But is there too much energy exhausting your fuel, or not enough energy tending it?

The third cycle of *The 49 Professions of Joy* redefines how you create encouragement and motivation. I do not want you to take that as an invitation to work yourself to death. Far from it. I want you to be fed and nourished by your activities, not consumed by them. These are not Professions of workaholism.

We build legacies with actions. Aspirations are air feeding your flame, but you must enact them. Whether you have too many or too few, write aspirations down. You can definitely have too much or too little going on in your head to let your body act. Keep some kind of recorded journal handy, whether it be written, typed, or audio recorded notes. Avoid puffing or snuffing your industrious fire out.

Feed: Consume, provide.

Collapsing supernova:

I make. I destroy.

# #15 OF 49

## I PROFESS THAT — I DO — EVERYTHING FROM THE INTENT OF BALANCE.

*MANIPURA: FIRE (I DO) TOUCHES MANIPURA: FIRE (I DO)*

Creation is duality, constantly cycling and recycling. Consider this: Everything constantly changes through dynamic balance, whether we can see it from our egocentric vantage point or not. At the personal level? No, it may not seem that everything balances at all. But taking the broader view? Yes, everything comes from and returns to the stuff of eternity. Remember **Profession #1**?

Feed is a word of note, because it takes contrasting meanings simultaneously, but two in particular. I need to feed the cat. I need to feed. One is sharing, the other ingesting. Feeding can be giving or receiving, or both simultaneously. Your work (hopefully) feeds your ambition, which then feeds your desire to continue achieving. This is a self-sustaining reward paradigm.

Stars are a great image here, because in consuming themselves they feed everything else. Even you eat sunlight. You ingest it as stored energy in food. Fusion, fission. Creating, deconstructing. Exploding out from its own heat, but collapsing in from its own gravity. Pushing itself apart, holding itself together.

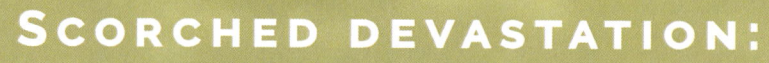

Scorched devastation:

Ravaged forests kindle growth.

Fecund, open, keen.

# #16 OF 49

## I PROFESS THAT — I DO — APPROPRIATE RECKONINGS OF MY RELATIONSHIPS.

*MANIPURA: FIRE (I DO)* TOUCHES *ANAHATA: WOOD (I LOVE)*

Wood is the heart chakra's Elemental, because plants weave rooted connections. From Anahata we project ourselves outward and forge relationships. But sometimes dangerous undergrowth accumulates in the forest. In **Profession #10** we looked at keeping your yard tidy. Here we have to consider more drastic landscaping measures.

Are you intertwined within nourishing, fulfilling relationships? If yes, awesome! (Check in with **Profession #8**, if you experience doubt.) If no . . .

I am not necessarily telling you to suddenly unleash your incendiary wrath in a policy of scorched earth. But when it's truly time for a reset, do it as compassionately as is appropriate (which might be not at all).

Wildfires destroy woods; however, that destruction feeds new growth. When is it necessary to protect your forest from conflagrations, and when is it necessary to burn it all away? Controlled fires are not bad. They provide nutrients and sky space for the next generation. Always preventing fires means the eventual burn will be devastating; however, always burning means never allowing new growth to take hold.

Incinerate lies,

ignite impotent breezes,

haul ideals aloft!

# #17 OF 49

## I PROFESS THAT — I DO — THAT WHICH I CLAIM, AND THAT WHICH I ADVISE.

*MANIPURA: FIRE (I DO) TOUCHES VISHUDHA: AIR (I SAY)*

Adding Fire (I DO) to Air (I SAY) causes the air to expand, creating lift. The image I got from this combination was hot air balloons or paper prayer lanterns. I think of this as putting action to words. For me that means practicing what you preach.

The sense here is that what we say about — or to — ourselves defines our values and ideals. Keeping faith with those makes us honest, reliable, and trustworthy. I avoided floating and soaring imagery in this haiku, because those are passive activities. Comfortably or lackadaisically riding wind thermals is exactly what I am advising you not to do.

We have to actively and purposefully propel and boost ourselves to reach our ideals. What happens if the balloon's fire dies? If our values don't require effort, they probably aren't very valuable.

Don't just be puffed up with words. Set a fire under your ass, and do what you promised yourself and others. Strive to share or pay forward toward the world's store of integrity.

Fluid potential's

boiling, percolating brew:

Effort's elixir.

# #18 OF 49

## I PROFESS THAT — I DO — IN THE WORLD WHAT I SEE IN MY MIND.

**MANIPURA: FIRE (I DO)** TOUCHES **AJÑA: WATER (I SEE)**

I work best when I have a deadline, or when pressed by some external source of accountability. As I write this, I know I have been holding up my graphic designer, and that embarrassment is the only reason I am doing this at all right now (my apologies, Christina!). Obviously I have a tendency to procrastinate. I mean, it took me 24 years to create the class for which I composed these haiku and Professions!

As I mentioned in my biography, I am evenly left brain/right brain dominant. Perhaps it's a coincidence, but I am also an evenly big picture/tiny details person. All this together seems to mean that I need to find a better balance between my internal artist and my internal editor.

This combination of Elementals addresses applying action (Fire) to knowledge (Water). Your many fluid ideas bubble up, but it's not enough to have inspired dreams or ambitions! You have to actually put them into externally functional and shared forms. Purposefully transform ingredients into elixirs.

*Related entry:* **Haiku #23**

Dawn's beaming hero:

Warrior — shift — Militant:

Noon's scorching villain.

# #19 OF 49

## I PROFESS THAT — I DO — WHAT I BELIEVE IS RIGHT WITHOUT FORGETTING WHAT IS GOOD.

**MANIPURA: FIRE (I DO)** TOUCHES **SAHASRARA: AKASHA (I KNOW)**

While considering fire in heaven, the obvious image was the sun itself. When contemplating the combination of doing and knowing, especially knowing from a spiritual perspective, I was taken with the idea of holy war: Putting faith into action.

Note specifically that "shift" perfectly balances the haiku. Structure's retrograde point: Warrior versus Militant. This shift could take countless forms, but in particular I mean perspective. And not necessarily your own. The fighter probably sees themselves as a warrior hero, but their rivals or victims likely see them as a militant villain. History and victors.

When you aggressively promote your beliefs, are you a dawn-like beaming hero warrior fighting for the good? Or have you shifted, and now you are a scorching noontime blazing militant? When you fight for what's "right," do you do it from a place of kindness and justice or cruelty and despotism? What is the shift? Do you always picture yourself heroically? Could your adversaries perceive you similarly, or only as a villain?

*Related entry:* **Haiku #46**

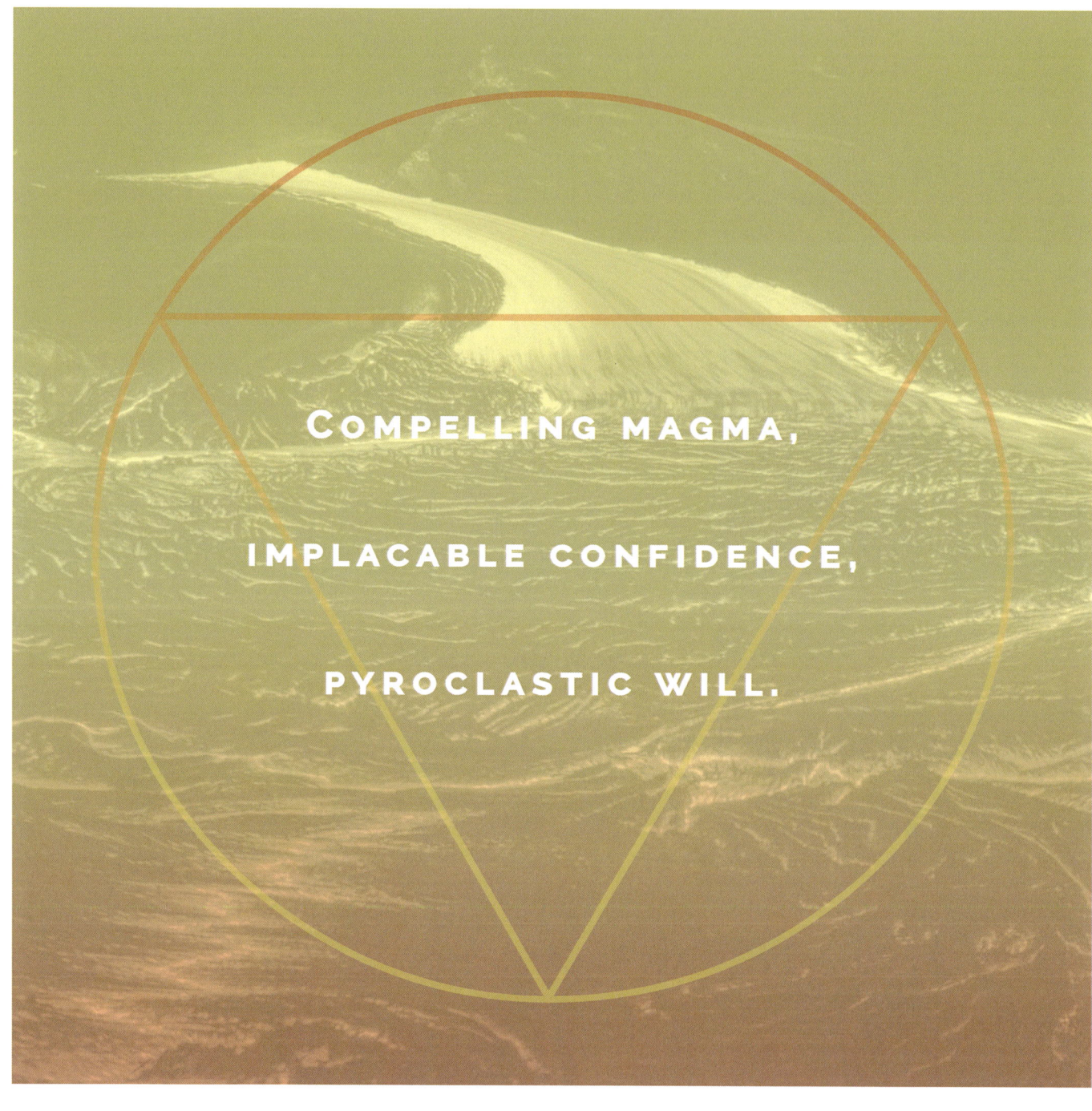

# #20 OF 49

## I PROFESS THAT — I DO — WITH RESOLVE THAT WHICH IS BEST FOR MY WELLBEING.

### MANIPURA: FIRE (I DO) TOUCHES MULADHARA: EARTH (I AM)

Fire and earth meld. Lava flows! Muladhara addresses self, safety, and sanity. The idea here is straightforward: Unapologetically make choices that keep you stable and healthy. Yes, there are times to put your own needs aside, but there are fundamentally critical situations where that option is off the table.

I have often had a hard time saying no. I have accepted any number of impositions (many irritating, some foolish, and a few devastating). I am not a better person for it. Many people will pursue Profession #20 like a military tactic. I am not telling you to be ruthless, fraudulent, or conniving. I am reminding you not to needlessly sacrifice yourself.

Have you ever seen footage of pyroclastic flows? Nothing can stop them. If you know that someone is doing something, or trying to convince you to do something, that is destructive to your body, mind, heart, or soul — you tell them NO!

If they have a problem with that, *give them my email address*. I will sort them out. Trust.

Fold, smash, cool, repeat.

Naïveté yields wisdom,

I become my sword.

# #21 OF 49

## I PROFESS THAT — I DO — THAT GRINDING WORK OF SELF-IMPROVEMENT.

### MANIPURA: FIRE (I DO) TOUCHES SVADISTHANA: METAL (I FEEL)

As a wellness coach and personal trainer, it is my task to help people forge their best version of themselves. I cannot do the work for them, but I can give them advice, encouragement, and accountability. I am a coach who always has a coach. It is an investment in my ongoing education. I have learned an extraordinary amount concerning what I want to do (and what I absolutely will not do) by watching others and better understanding myself.

I see only two reasons to ask for someone's advice: 1) You want to accomplish something similar to what they have done, or 2) You want to avoid what you perceive as their mistakes. Good manners and prudence dictate you not tell them which is on your mind.

In **Profession #3** you were the architect and mason, in **#10** the gardener. In **#38** you will be the potter. Here you are the blacksmith. You must create your own reality. Imagine how keen your blade is after so many grinding experiences!

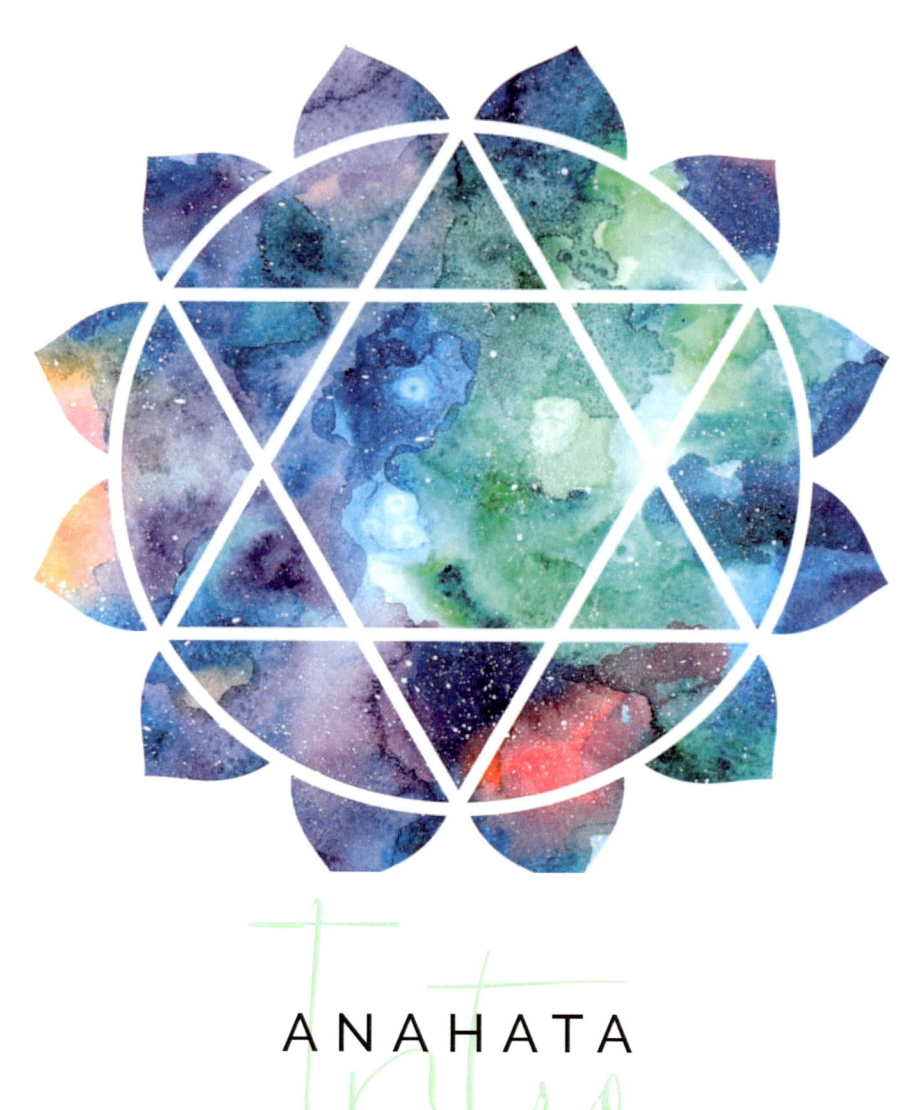

**COLOR**
GREEN

**ELEMENTAL**
WOOD

**PURPOSE**
CONNECTING

**MANTRA**
"I LOVE"

ANAHATA
*Intro*

Also called the Heart Chakra, this energy vortex is located in the center of your chest beside your heart. This is the halfway point, connecting and balancing your physical chakras with your metaphysical chakras. It is the intersection: By its nature it is our source of connectivity within and between ourselves and each other. This "I LOVE" is not the English idea of love, but rather resembles the Classical Greek. There is love of self; romantic love; patriotism; friendship, family, neighborliness, and community fellowship; loyalty; and many other types of connection. When it is healthy and aligned you will share harmony. Cooperation, friendship, collaboration, and appreciation are life's blood flowing from your heart. They grow gradually, putting out roots, tangling each other in a thicket of interdependence.

When it is misaligned your sprouts are stunted by isolation, hatred, jealousy, and ingratitude. But is there too much energy feeding choking weeds, or not enough energy withering your budding flowers?

The fourth cycle of *The 49 Professions of Joy* redefines how you form bonds. As I said before, this goes beyond dating and marriage. This is the tree bearing fruit. That includes empathy, compassion, and encouragement. This is generosity in all its forms.

There are millions of plant species, and endless ways we touch each other. We ourselves are the network. There are not only rose bushes, fruit trees, and gorgeous Japanese maples. There are weeds, vines, and brambles. Some flowers are beautiful but toxic: Beware the daffodils growing in your garden.

Tangled, grasping knots:

Deep roots anchor our shared fate.

Billions live. One life.

# #22 OF 49

## I PROFESS THAT — I LOVE — MY LIFE, AND THAT THE WORLD IS A BETTER PLACE WITH ME IN IT.

### ANAHATA: WOOD (I LOVE) TOUCHES ANAHATA: WOOD (I LOVE)

The Anahata series is about connection and relationships, and for this reason it should be no surprise that the haiku in this series overlap with each other in many interesting ways. That is the very nature of this chakra.

If you have worked with dirt, you know how complex plants' root systems are. It can become difficult or impossible to unsnarl them from each other. Many types of plants cast entire networks from one individual. This creates what looks like separate individuals at a distance. Try to remove them, and you find that they are arms connected to a single subterranean body. What might appear to be dozens of trees in a thicket can actually be one tree that has put up a cluster of trunks.

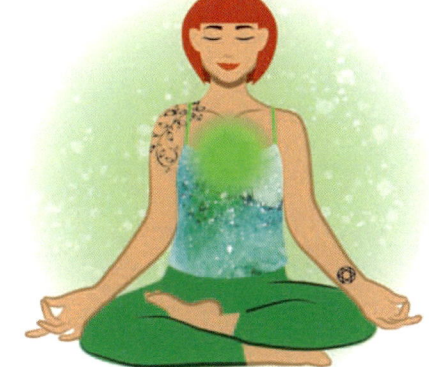

This is how I see people. It may look like we are isolated individuals, but we form networks. We affect each other at every level, and should value every leaf on our tree.

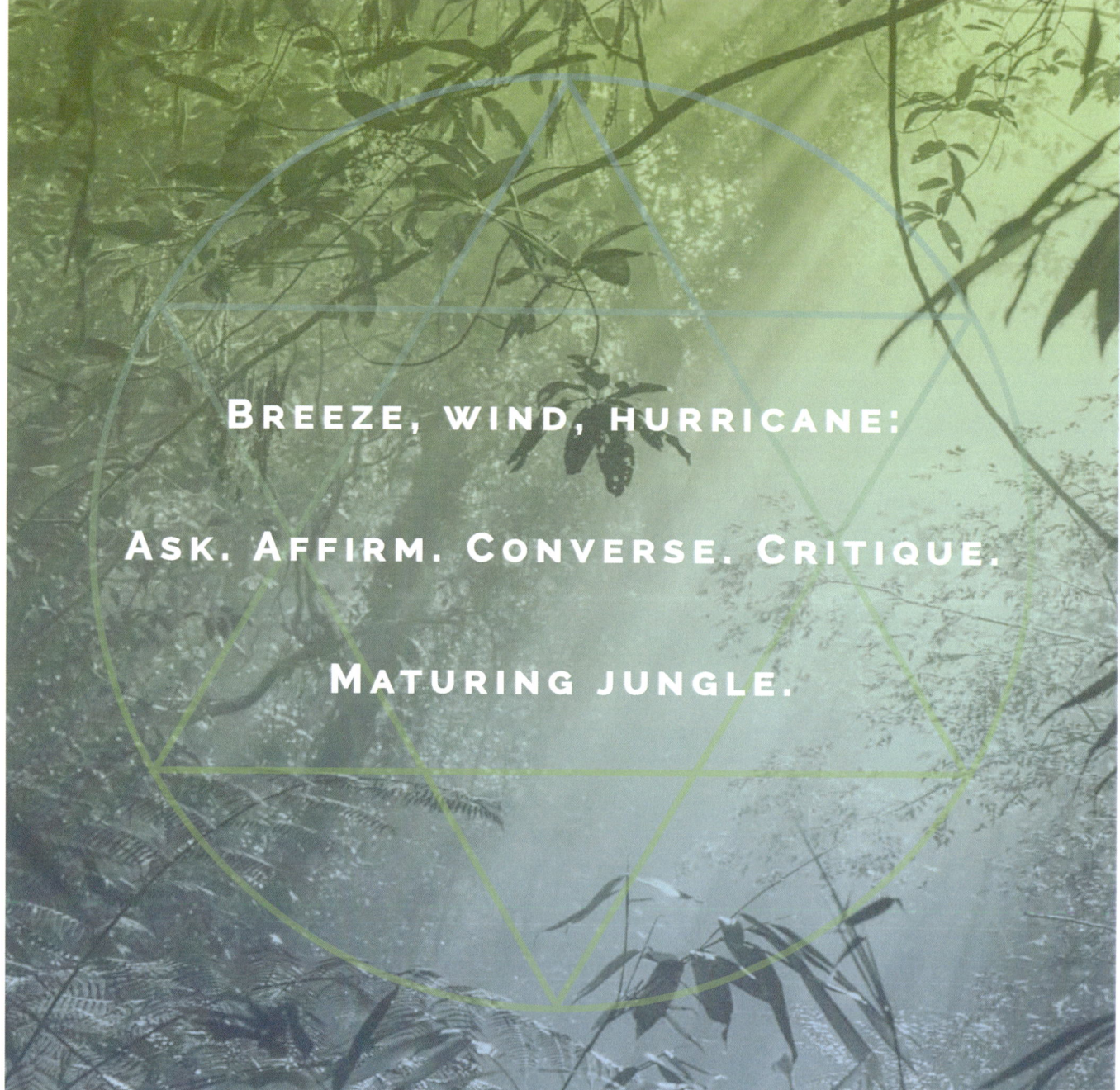

# #23 OF 49

## I PROFESS THAT — I LOVE — EXPERIENCING A WIDE VARIETY OF PERSPECTIVES.

*ANAHATA: WOOD (I LOVE) TOUCHES VISHUDHA: AIR (I SAY)*

The Elementals Wood and Air commingle conceptually like plants do literally when they absorb oxygen. Respiration's chemical process deconstructs the sugar created during photosynthesis, releasing solar power the plants initially captured. This is the energy plants use specifically to grow. Notice that Professions #23 (respiration), #24 (capillarity), and #28 (photosynthesis) work together as a set, using the metaphor of plant growth to contemplate healthy socializing.

We access exuberant energy and excitement derived from family, friends, supporters, and colleagues by maintaining dialogues with them. When we laugh, joke, sing, play, talk, reminisce, and collaborate, we feed off the enthusiasm they supply, breaking it down to power our own personal growth. Their conversations help us mature by way of discussion, debate, affirmations, and constructive criticisms. Those discussions can be breezy or stormy. We need to share ideas, just as plants need oxygen. It breathes fresh air into us.

Note that #41 also touches on collaboration: The phase when we gather ideas before discussing them. Remember from #18 that you must enact your ideas.

Eden's tree imbibes insight. Roots grasp truth's vision, slaking heartened thirst.

# #24 OF 49

## I PROFESS THAT — I LOVE — LEARNING, ESPECIALLY FROM THE WISDOM OF OTHERS.

*ANAHATA: WOOD (I LOVE)* TOUCHES *AJÑA: WATER (I SEE)*

It makes sense that many haiku in the Anahata series tangle together. Connections are defined by interactions, and the branches of these poems' ideas weave together to create a sense of constant sharing. Notice that Professions *#23* (respiration), #24 (capillarity), and *#28* (photosynthesis) work together as a set, using the metaphor of plant growth to contemplate healthy socializing.

Trees draw water into themselves as part of the process of releasing the energy required for growing. Learning (represented here by drinking) is growing. This particular haiku is not about the important lessons we learn on our own, but those we receive from teachers, coaches, mentors, and scholars.

Roots grasp and delve into the heart of the matter, drawing thirstily at the knowledge that flows in from a network of ideas and inspiration, heartening a deep love of and connection to truth. This tree of knowledge grows in a paradise of curiosity. In this garden, knowledge is not tainting or sinful, it is satiating our need for intellectual, imaginative freedom.

Striving heavenward,

our human forest cradles

diverse, supple trees.

# #25 OF 49

## I PROFESS THAT — I LOVE — A WIDE VARIETY OF PEOPLE AND THE RICHNESS THEIR DIVERSITY ADDS TO THE WORLD.

*ANAHATA: WOOD (I LOVE)* TOUCHES *SAHASRARA: AKASHA (I KNOW)*

Sahasrara amplifies any image's sense of expansiveness: So then, the world's sacred grove. When love comes from a place of universal acceptance, tribalism must fall away. We, the individual saplings who populate the forest of humanity, are as varied and unique as each tree in a woodland. We are hardy survivors who bend and adapt.

By extending inclusion to all, we make the whole coppice stronger, more resilient. The arc of history finds us *slowly* reaching upward toward ideals like international cooperation and alliance. Brambles like bigotry and isolationism are *gradually* being shaded out by this canopy. Like mixed forests, we can retain our individuality while growing next to others not like ourselves.

My cautionary tale about disconnection: As a self-isolating introvert, Bipolar II disorder undermines *everything*. I retreated for years into my apartment-sanctuary, and seclusion became my default. Now I have to consciously and persistently resist family history: Our men become antisocial recluses with age. I do not want this.

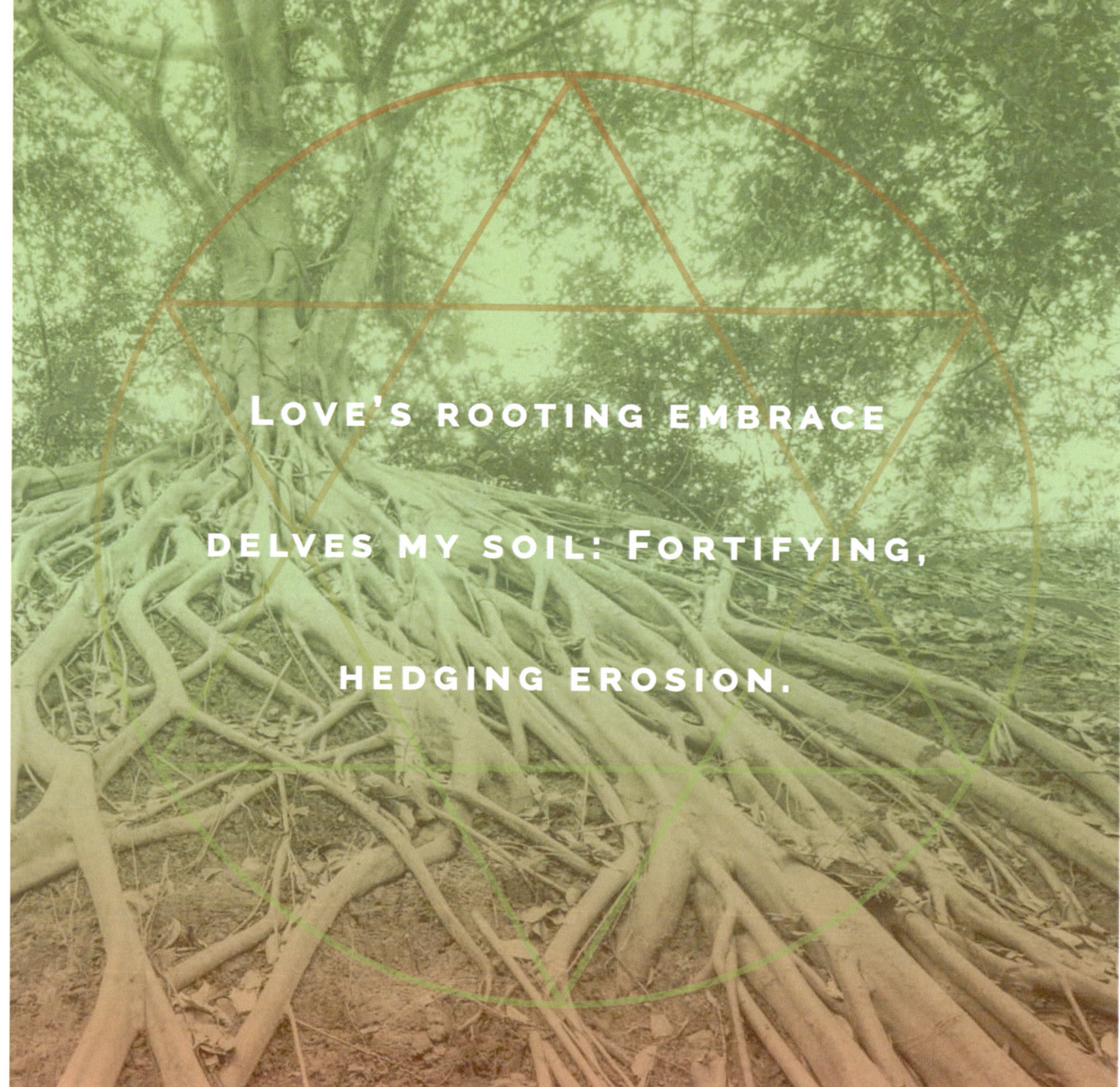

Love's rooting embrace delves my soil: Fortifying, hedging erosion.

# #26 OF 49

## I PROFESS THAT — I LOVE — AND APPRECIATE THOSE WHO HELP ME TO REMAIN STABLE.

*ANAHATA: WOOD (I LOVE) TOUCHES MULADHARA: EARTH (I AM)*

How does Wood affect Earth? Plants penetrate downward, holding dirt intact. A lack of roots allows for erosion. That was literal. I mean it figuratively: A lack of connection undermines your wellness. We need other people.

Love and connection affect your well-being, health, safety, and stability by holding it all together. When you are worn down, do you have a network of people who help you build back up? Do you help others when they need it?

Relationships hold us in place psychologically and emotionally, but they survive only when rooted into rich soil that nourishes them in return. You are the soil that feeds your relationships. It is you who encourages the roots to delve. You help them, which helps you keep your foundation. In a healthy relationship people can expect the same in return.

In the haiku, "rooting" and "hedge" are nods to plants. Although rooting is both a way of embracing or stabilizing, it is also a way of encouraging: I am rooting for you!

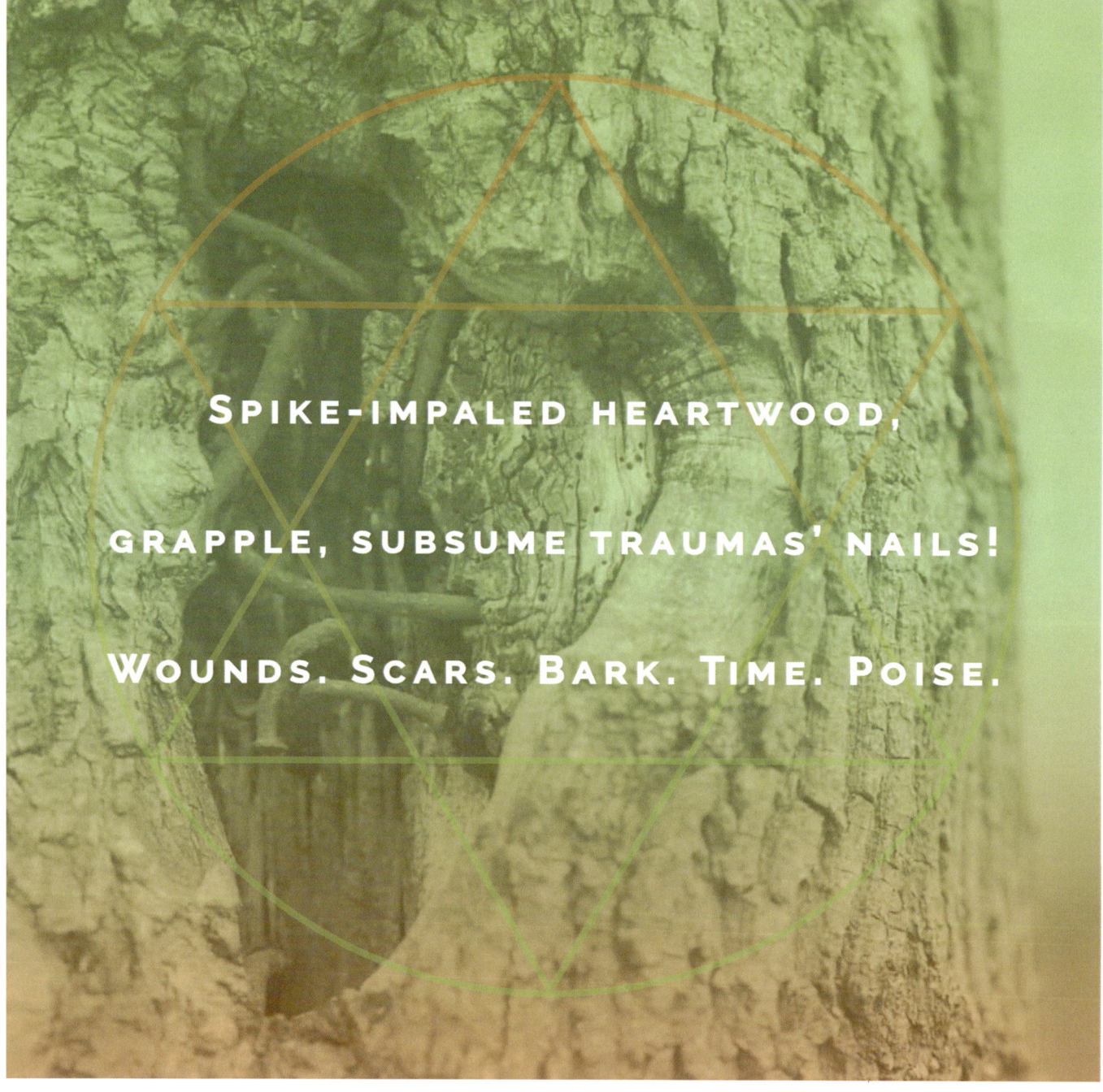

Spike-impaled heartwood,

grapple, subsume traumas' nails!

Wounds. Scars. Bark. Time. Poise.

# #27 OF 49

## I PROFESS THAT — I LOVE — ALL MY EXPERIENCES, BECAUSE THEY HAVE MADE ME STRONGER.

### ANAHATA: WOOD (I LOVE) TOUCHES SVADISTHANA: METAL (I FEEL)

Some relationships are hurtful, scarring. When I was considering how Metal affects Wood, all the images kept coming back to chainsaws obliterating jungles. I have had very bad luck in love. So perhaps that is my own trauma vibrating out from my chakras. Although I try to avoid negativity, sometimes I just need to vent.

Arborglyphs are marks left in tree bark when people carve it. Often you will see anonymous people declaring their love. That is what I wanted to examine: The marks love etches into us. Another interesting phenomenon is how trees will grow around and eventually swallow nails. I have a picture from a trip to Portland, OR of a tree devouring a fire hydrant. True story!

At any rate, we are resilient, and we heal around our injuries. Chops, cuts, slashes, punctures — all are buried in our flesh, heart, and mind. But we can still thrive and grow, eventually bearing our faded scars as we stand tall and grow ever stronger.

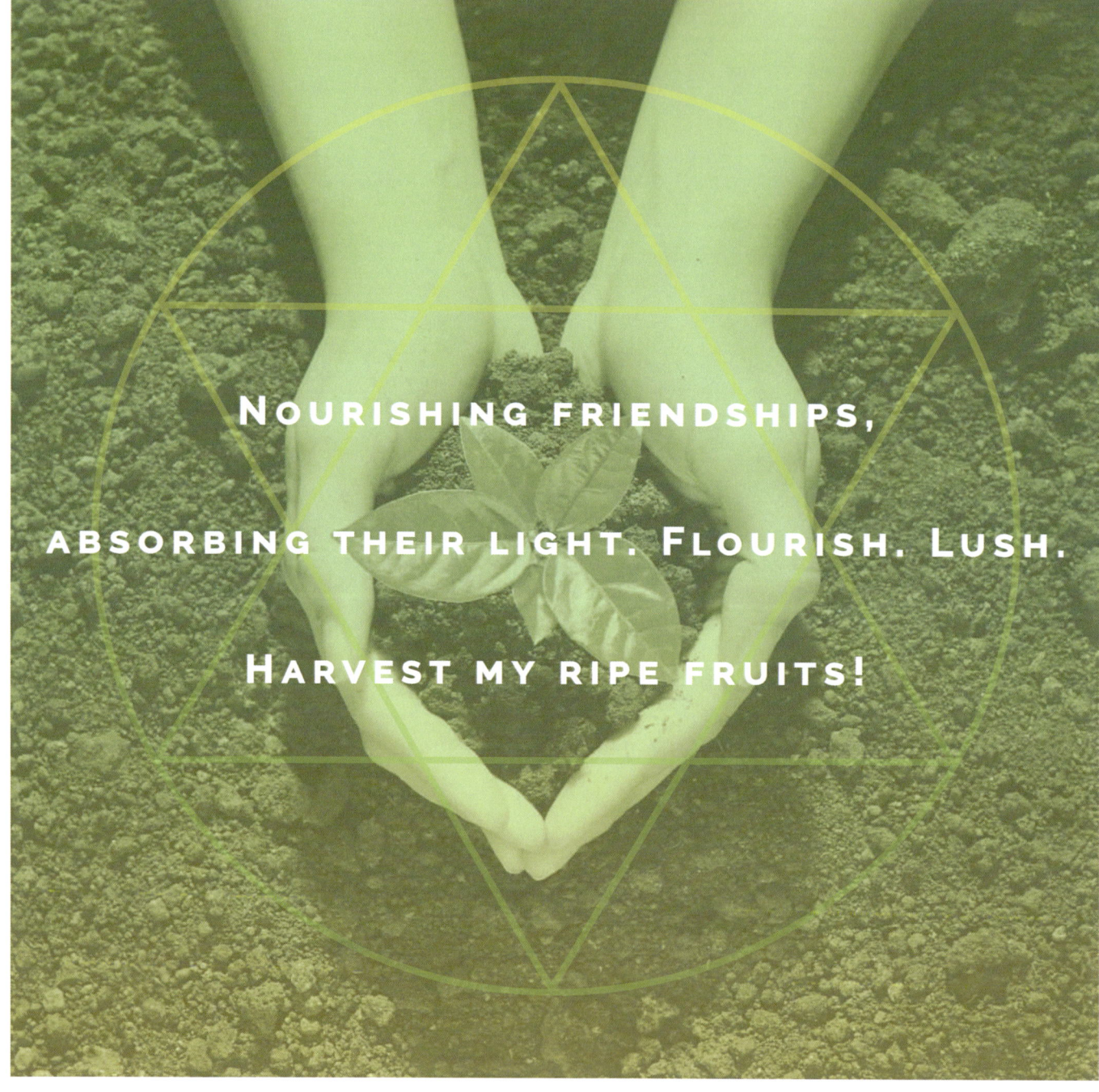

# #28 OF 49

## I PROFESS THAT — I LOVE — TO GIVE AND RECEIVE GENEROUS, THRIVING ENERGY.

**ANAHATA: WOOD (I LOVE)** TOUCHES **MANIPURA: FIRE (I DO)**

Wood meets Fire is definitely not the same as Fire meets Wood. In **Profession #16** we needed to clear out unhealthy relationships. Here we're basking in the light of good ones! Notice that **Professions #23** (respiration), **#24** (capillarity), and #28 (photosynthesis) work together as a set, using the metaphor of plant growth to contemplate healthy socializing.

How do healthy connections affect our actions? People whose light energizes us will be encouraging and animating. They will refuel our need to succeed and thrive. They help us move forward toward goals. From my loved ones, I absorb their warmth and turn it into the energy that feeds my ambition. Their light becomes my own, and I feed others with my actions as well.

The energy you gratefully absorb powers photosynthesis. The energy you generously share is fruit. You are nourished and you are nourishing. You get opportunity, you share the fruits of your labor. Just as captured sunlight is the source of food energy, love is the source of accomplishment.

*Related entry:* **Haiku #6**

**COLOR**
AQUA

**ELEMENTAL**
AIR

**PURPOSE**
EXPRESSING

**MANTRA**
"I SAY"

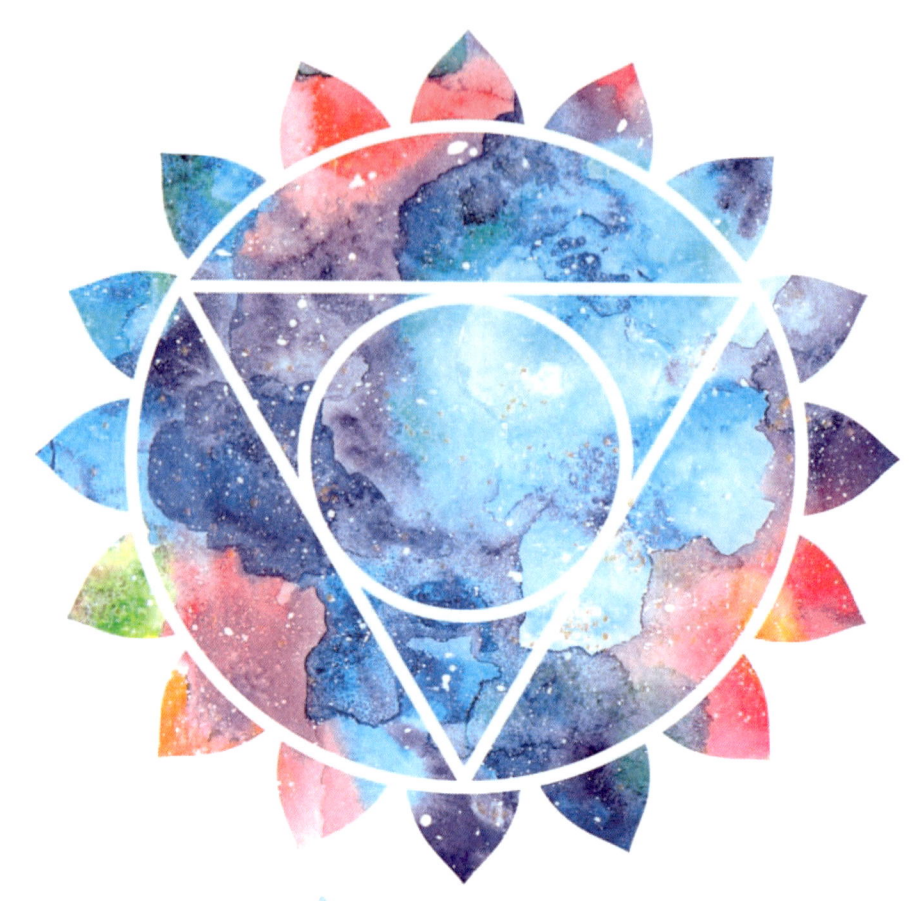

VISHUDHA

Also called the Throat Chakra, this energy vortex is located in your throat. If you consider that what you say can breathe new life into a conversation, you will understand the connection to the Air Elemental. But let us not restrict "I SAY" to only the words we utter. You express yourself in many ways, both verbally and nonverbally. Your body language, facial expressions, and tone of voice carry meaning. Words you write are not always read aloud. Poetry, art, music, dance, and all forms of creativity allow you to express yourself. When it is healthy and aligned you will communicate clearly. Inspiration, communication, clarity, and motivation can all float on the breezes you blow from your mouth.

When it is misaligned your words become gales of discouragement, confusion, censorship, or conflict. But is there too much energy spinning out hurricanes, or not enough energy stagnating each breath?

The fifth cycle of *The 49 Professions of Joy* redefines how you express ideas. Do you have conversations or exchange concepts efficiently and productively? Do you interrupt or dominate others? Avoid gossip. Bullying injures everyone involved. Create the art that contextualizes your ideas. How do you get past writer's block?

This "sticks and stones" comparison with words is entirely inaccurate, and frankly ignorant. The idea that "words will never harm me," is essentially a lie unto itself. That is a dysfunction within our culture's collective Vishudha experience. Words are not meaningless. They are extraordinarily powerful. Denying this invites and sustains energetic imbalances.

# Heaving, writhing winds:

# Self-inflicted tornadoes?

# Whirling dervishes?

# #29 OF 49

## I PROFESS THAT — I SAY — TRUTH KINDLY AND KINDNESS TRUTHFULLY, ESPECIALLY TO MYSELF.

*VISHUDHA: AIR (I SAY) TOUCHES VISHUDHA: AIR (I SAY)*

The Vishudha sequence begins with the way Air affects itself. In my mind it begins rushing and whirling, becoming stronger while creating a vortex. Imagine it as repeating ineffectual words while also twisting them into something other than what they were. In politics or media this is spin. These statements often create whirlwinds of drama and controversy. Hence blowback, resulting in yet more comments that convince no one of anything.

And when this is turned inward? You might feel yourself spinning out of control when you repeat the same insults toward yourself ad nauseam. Be aware how you often build and magnify the damage from hurtful, unhelpful statements. Perhaps consider using your inner voice to chant a repetitious mantra that transports you to a place of twirling peace? Find videos of whirling dervishes.

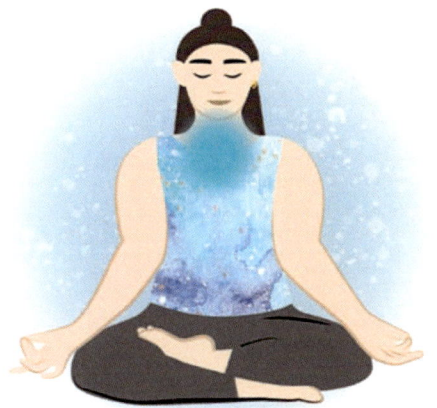

If there is a hard truth you must tell, as in *Profession #35*, do it compassionately where possible. But while you are being kind, make sure you are being honest. Healthy people do not appreciate empty flattery.

Undulating sea:

Headwinds, crosswinds, tailwinds gust.

Surge, roiling tempest!

# #30 OF 49

## I PROFESS THAT — I SAY — MY IDEAS, AND WELCOME OTHERS TO SCRUTINIZE THEM.

### VISHUDHA: AIR (I SAY) TOUCHES AJÑA: WATER (I SEE)

Air touching Water has to be waves. It cannot be anything else, can it? The imagery is just too obvious. Think about all the different types of waves though: From tiny capillary waves, all the way up to infragravity waves!

As wind moves across the surface of lakes and oceans it creates the dynamic, fluid action happening before our literal eyes. Similarly, a person's expressions or views can make waves, because their ideas have moved what other people know behind their Third Eyes.

Think about the excited discussions, vigorous debates, stormy arguments, and funny jokes that have made you reconsider what you know. What about observations in art, poetry, prose, or drama that have changed the way you think, or shifted the way you understand the world?

Headwinds: How has what you said or read pushed back against or challenged your perspectives? Crosswinds: Has anyone ever blown you over, forcing you to totally rethink your opinions? Tailwinds: When have people confirmed or validated your ideas and propelled you forward?

*Related entry:* **Haiku #42**

Awed fascination:

Eternity's spectacle.

We gasped! Gratitude.

# #31 OF 49

## I PROFESS THAT — I SAY — CONTEMPLATIVE WORDS CONCERNING MY PLACE IN THE UNIVERSE.

*VISHUDHA: AIR (I SAY) TOUCHES SAHASRARA: AKASHA (I KNOW)*

Putting I SAY with I KNOW creates religion and philosophy. Akasha is the Elemental of "All," and its influence highlights the ethereal quality of a chakra. If Air is like the sky, then sky plus spirit is heaven, and words spoken to heaven are prayer.

There is a ubiquitous need for people to express wonder toward creation. Every culture tells stories to explain it and our place or purpose within it. That might express itself as prayer, mythology, sermons, research, lectures, or debates. Regardless of whether it be religious rituals, philosophical debates, or scientific hypotheses, we have always used words to explore and attempt to define or understand the eternal within which we find ourselves.

Whether you are a religious person or not, contemplating or dedicating some portion of your discussions toward your sense of purpose affords opportunities to understand the ways in which you can appreciate your life. Express wonder as you see best. I personally do not feel science contradicts spirituality. It is simply another language explaining universal principles.

Innuendos waft,

rippling sand, mutating dunes:

Relentless whispers.

# #32 OF 49

## I PROFESS THAT — I SAY — KIND WORDS TO AND ABOUT OTHER PEOPLE.

*VISHUDHA: AIR (I SAY)* TOUCHES *MULADHARA: EARTH (I AM)*

Let us consider how what you say (Air) affects someone's sense of health, wellbeing, or safety (Earth). Be mindful of comments you make that may be warping someone's experience of self or security. I think of people's feelings as being more akin to sand dunes than mountains, the winds of conversation constantly shifting and reforming them.

Gossip is a form of bullying. Period. Callous, careless, or insensitive comments can create far reaching, profound implications. What you perceive to be a passing observation might reshape someone else's life, causing huge dust-ups within them. The words you say or share affect other people's inner landscapes. I speak from first hand experience: Humiliation, insults, threats, and lies inflict lifelong torment.

It took many years (and I still struggle sometimes), but I no longer constantly feel I am disappearing into a sandpit trap. Psychologically it seemed like no matter how much I tried to climb out, I would tumble down the loose sides and smother in an avalanche of verbal debris.

Avoid causing that.

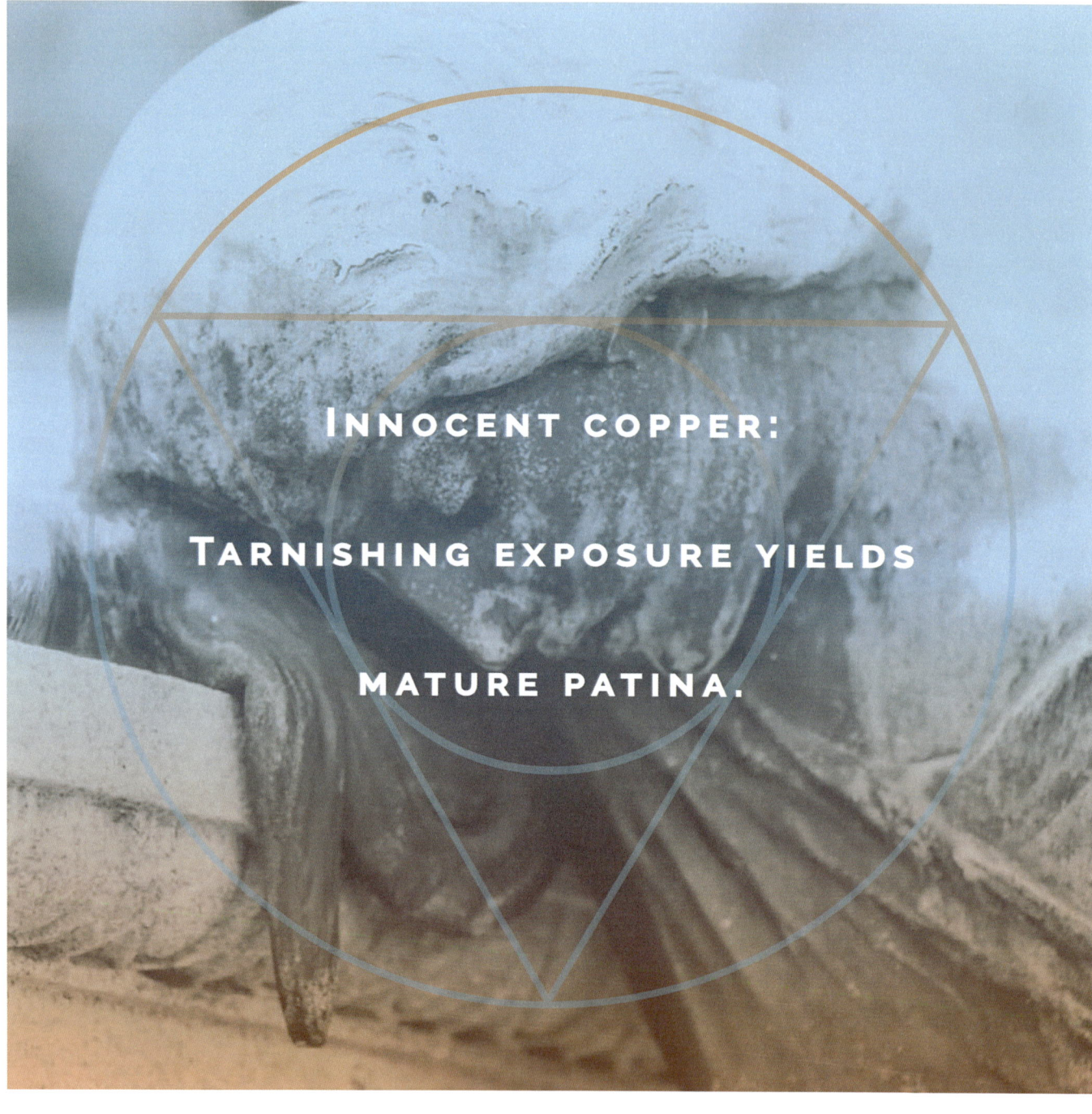

# #33 OF 49

## I PROFESS THAT — I SAY — WHAT I FEEL, KNOWING THAT SHARING IT WILL HELP ME TO MATURE.

### VISHUDHA: AIR (I SAY) TOUCHES SVADISTHANA: METAL (I FEEL)

In my mind, Air affecting Metal initially conjured images of corrosion. However, rather than thinking in terms of it being destructive, I prefer to think of it as being curative.

Expressing your feelings should not be the same as iron rusting. I definitely prefer to compare it to the patina on copper. **Profession #39** (Water touches Metal) addresses jealousy. For now, I want to consider emotional availability and honesty.

We cannot gain what we want or need emotionally if we never express or define it. Might we often be rebuffed? Sure. Will our requests or offers for emotional intimacy sometimes be rejected? I hope so: It teaches us how to polish our self esteem when it gets a little smudged by disappointment. But you will never get what truly gratifies your needs if you never discuss it.

These conversations expose us to the weathering influence of experience. It may be that we become less shiny, but we become able to express burnished dignity that evokes emotional wisdom.

Raging inferno:

Frenzied incineration?

Zephyr: Whispered spark.

# #34 OF 49

## I PROFESS THAT — I SAY — MY WORDS IN THE SPIRIT OF INSPIRING OTHERS TO GOODNESS.

### VISHUDHA: AIR (I SAY) TOUCHES MANIPURA: FIRE (I DO)

I have said repeatedly how powerful words are. If you doubt it, consider the way leaders use speeches. Gifted and persuasive orators throughout history have inflamed entire nations with their communication skills. Think of the profound influence of the glowing speeches by Abraham Lincoln, Franklin D. Roosevelt, Mahatma Gandhi, Winston Churchill, Martin Luther King, Jr., Maya Angelou, Nelson Mandela, and Barack Obama.

What about the shining beauty conjured by brilliant poets like Rumi, Khalil Gibran, Charles Baudelaire, Walt Whitman, and Emily Dickinson? Or the burning wit of Benjamin Franklin, Oscar Wilde, and David Sedaris?

And please never underestimate the awesome and terrible power of fear mongering and hate speech to ignite people to ruin: Robespierre, Marx, Hitler, Stalin, Mao, Osama bin Ladin, Idi Amin . . .

Your statements are powerful. What you say matters. Do you use your voice to hurt, anger, or inflame others? Or do you seek to inspire, soothe, and warm? What you say, no matter what medium or format, casts light into the world. What color is it?

*Related entry:* **Haiku #46**

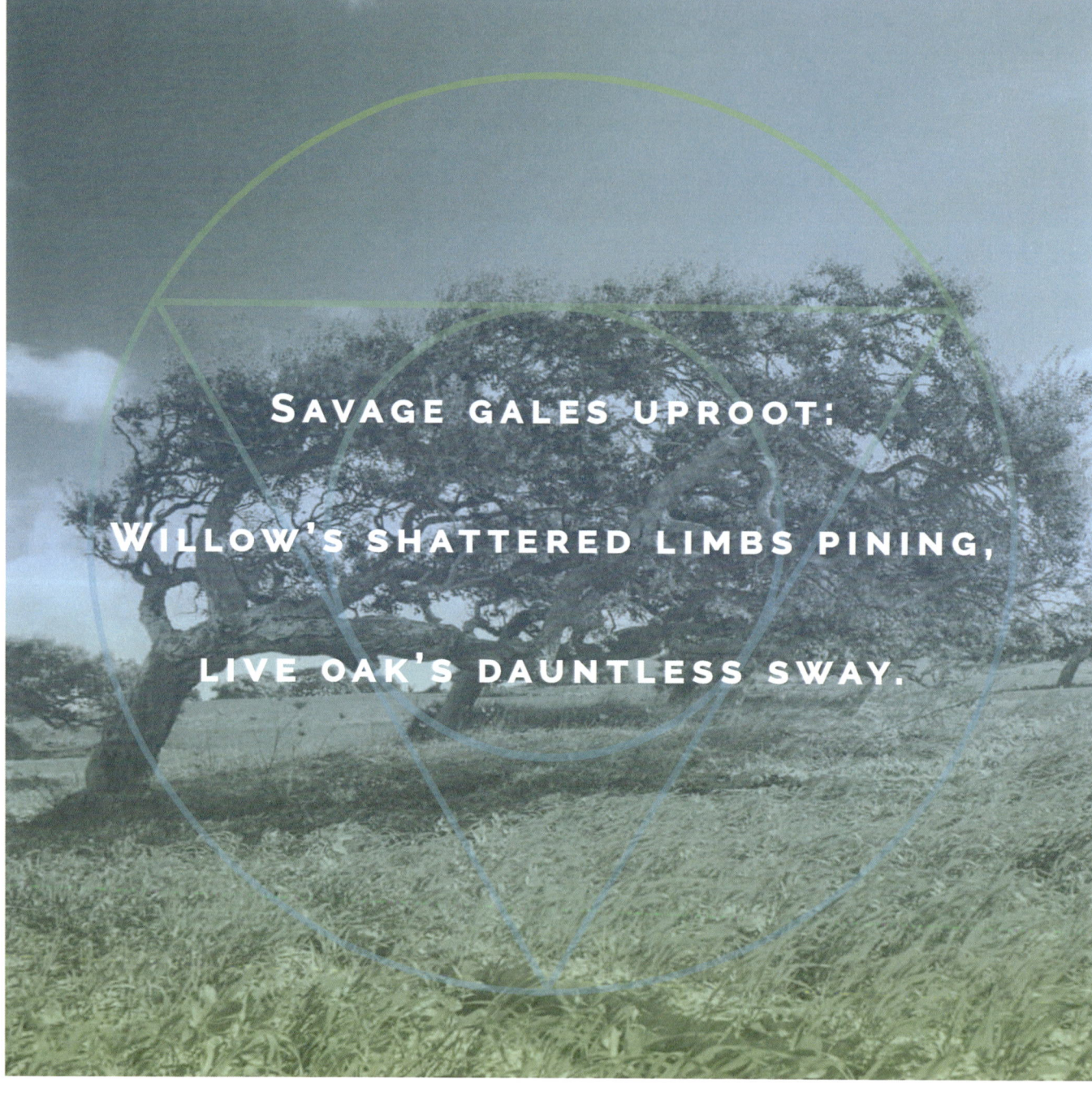

# #35 OF 49

## I PROFESS THAT — I SAY — WHAT WILL HELP ME AND OTHERS TO GROW.

*VISHUDHA: AIR (I SAY)* TOUCHES *ANAHATA: WOOD (I LOVE)*

*Them: "You can't take constructive criticism!" Me: "Perhaps you don't know how to give it."*

Criticism is tricky. But is it helpful to ignore it because it knocks us over sometimes? Should we be mindful how we give and receive feedback? See *Profession #29*. Cruelty, sarcasm, and rudeness are unnecessary.

Does it feel like harsh words will snap our branches? Sometimes. But criticism also forces us to adapt. Hopefully it doesn't leave us misshapen or permanently twisted. But the point here is not that we choose whether or not winds batter us. Consider rather whether we break or bend under their force.

I am not suggesting that you embrace cold stoicism, but that you remember to catch some of the wind in your leaves while letting the rest pass through. Grasp only gusts of feedback that are helpful. Let the rest blow away.

As a side note: I like the word play on "pining," because pine trees are vulnerable to strong winds, but they regrow relatively quickly.

**COLOR**
BLUE

**ELEMENTAL**
WATER

**PURPOSE**
KNOWING

**MANTRA**
"I SEE"

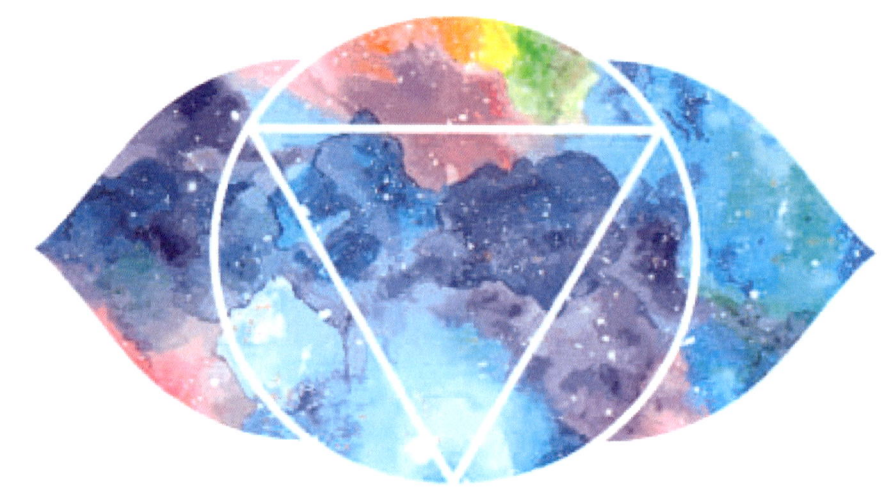

AJÑA

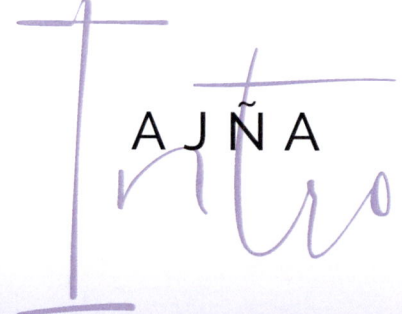

Also called the Third Eye or Brow Chakra, this energy vortex is located between your eyes. In the languages I speak and study, I have noticed consistently that "I SEE" is essentially interchangeable with "I KNOW" and/or "I UNDERSTAND." Consider not just that you see with your physical eyes, but also with your wisdom and intellect. Someone makes an assertion and/or demonstration, and you reply, "I see what you're saying and/or doing." Or another, "I will believe it when I see it." The literal and the conceptual are tied together. Entire oceans of knowledge are waiting to be delved. When Ajña is healthy and aligned you will understand openly. Perception, learning, curiosity, and invention flow through your open mind as you look with curious eyes at the worlds within and around you.

When it is misaligned you drown wisdom in presumption, ignorance, stubbornness, and dogma. But is there too much energy flooding into your mind, or not enough energy desiccating your inspiration?

The sixth cycle of *The 49 Professions of Joy* redefines how you embrace knowledge. Are you open to new ideas? Are you curious and intellectually nimble? How do you respond when someone or something interrupts what you thought you knew?

There are many ways of seeing, both literally and figuratively. With your physical eyes, explore the nuances between diffuse, focused, honed, and keen gazes. What do you learn from each? Alternatively, these concepts translate directly to the amount of interest you put into new topics.

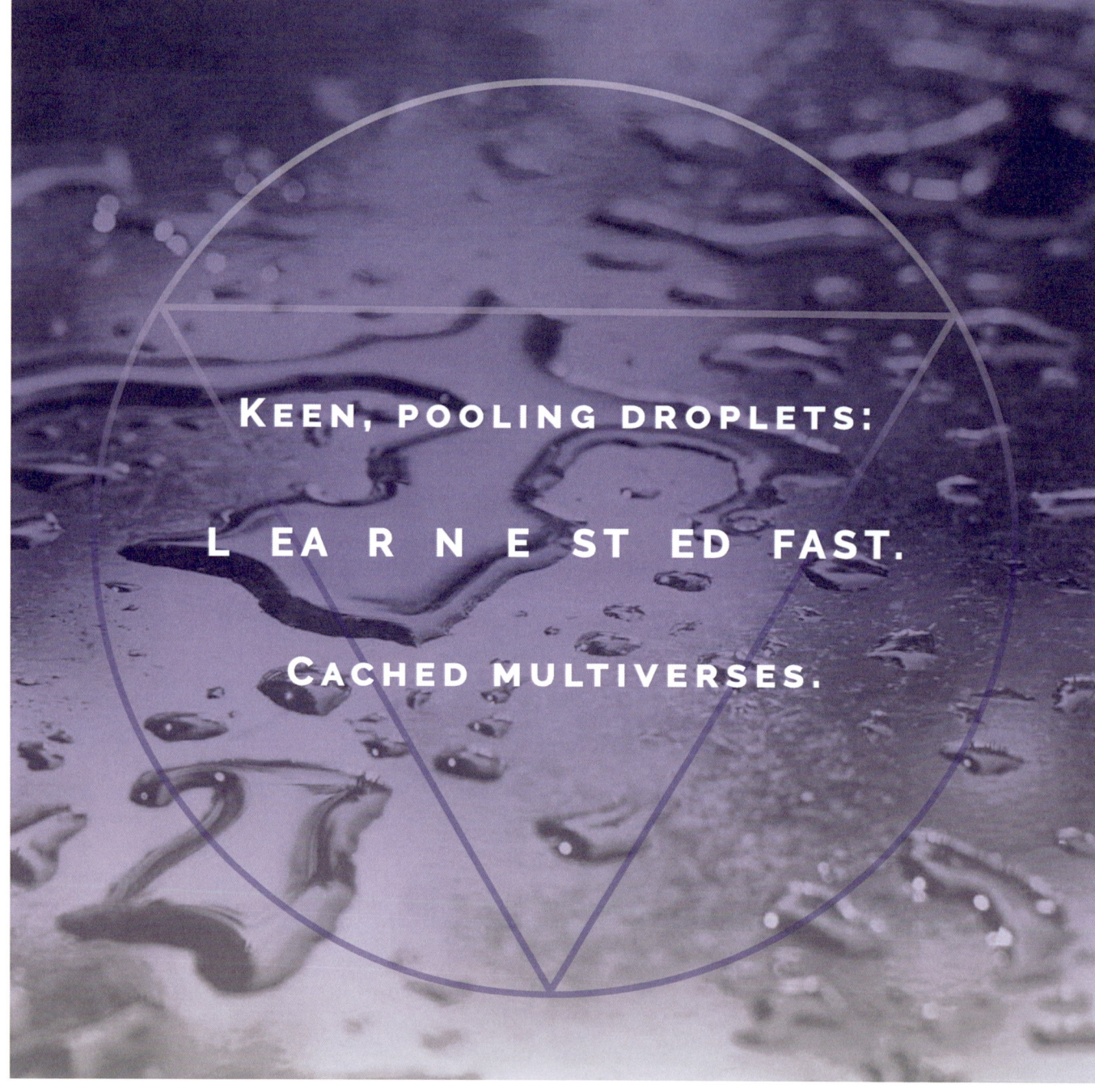

# #36 OF 49

## I PROFESS THAT — I SEE — MYSELF AS A CURIOUS CHILD ASKING ONE THOUSAND TIMES, "WHY?"

*AJÑA: WATER (I SEE)* TOUCHES *AJÑA: WATER (I SEE)*

For Ajña, seeing resembles understanding. When Water touches Water, it conjoins. But it can still change shape and become gas, liquid, or solid.

To LEARN begets learning. When one question is answered, it leads to more questions. We are the child who asks the EARNEST, unrelenting, "Why?" Every answer needs another, with worlds NESTED within worlds.

Knowledge grabs onto itself in all directions, pooling deep oceans of thought. Droplets are STEDFAST as they do this by way of adhesion: The molecules attract each other. Facts also cling together, meaning the more we learn, the more we know.

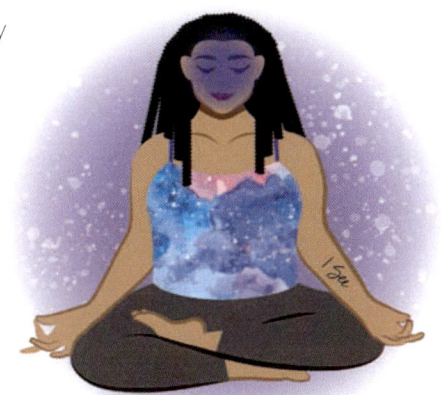

Swim in your pool of curiosity. Watch it expand in every direction. Learning is the water filling the changing shape of your mind, and it can take all forms: Imagination (gas), consideration (liquid), and invention (solid).

Speaking of droplets grabbing onto each other: LEARN, EARNEST, NESTED, STEDFAST (yes, it's seven syllables). I am really quite smitten by this haiku. If any demanded cleverness, it was #36.

Sorrow's drowning thirst.

Ecstatic dissolution,

quench my parched spirit!

# #37 OF 49

## I PROFESS THAT — I SEE — THAT I WANT TO SEE MORE.

### *AJÑA: WATER (I SEE)* TOUCHES *SAHASRARA: AKASHA (I KNOW)*

When Water connects to Akasha, the divine nature of knowledge becomes spiritual acceptance. Something like faith, but not as rigid as dogma. Deeper understanding leads a soul toward the infinite and/or divine.

Many cultures see water as a holy substance used in various ways to cleanse something not only physically, but also spiritually. Baptism, perhaps the most familiar version of this in the West, is a sacrament used to wash the soul of sin and to bring a person into their faith community.

In other cultures, water imbues knowledge, affects rain, washes ritual objects, improves vision, etc. Seeking understanding of Self and one's context within the universe is often called metaphorical thirst.

Dissolution has multiple, simultaneous readings. All of them are relevant and valid. This includes the spiritual elation achieved in some religions during boisterous festivals or ecstatic rituals of wanton, unfettered indulgence. These practices view the profane, excessive, bawdy, and sensuous as having particular sanctity of their own. In this, perhaps we allow wine to be water's metaphysical cousin?

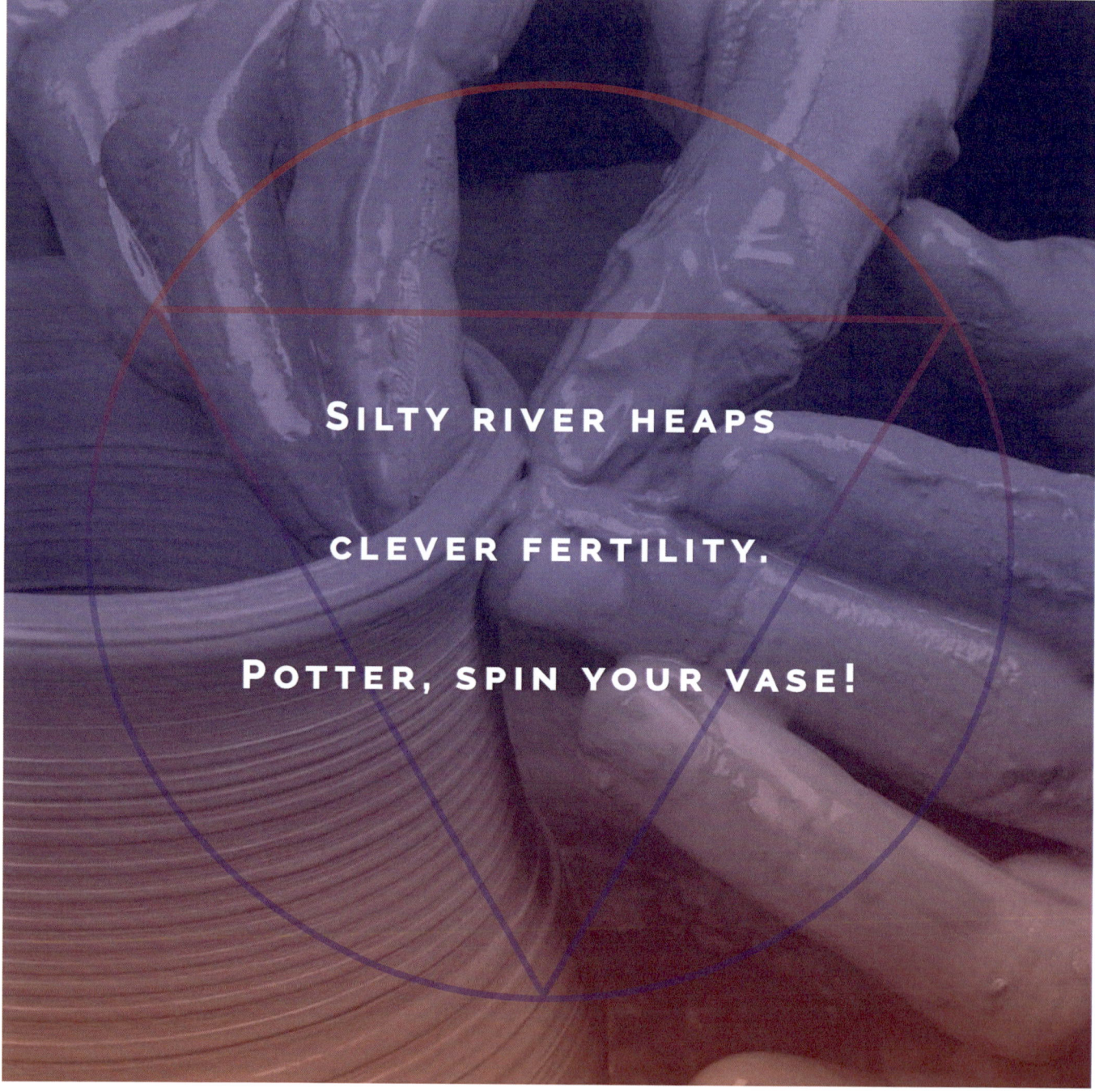

# #38 OF 49

## I PROFESS THAT — I SEE — THE INHERENT VALUE IN LEARNING AS I ENVISION SHAPING MY LIFE.

### AJÑA: WATER (I SEE) TOUCHES MULADHARA: EARTH (I AM)

Spongy brains literally function better than dryer ones. Water makes Earth a tool of creation, both as fertile soil and as malleable clay. With knowledge, training, and education come a better chance of realizing not only what one wants to be, but also how to accomplish it. Know thyself, yes?

Fertile river silt allowed entire civilizations to thrive as they learned to cultivate crops and then develop other new innovations. Similarly, potters can use their skill to pull useful and/or beautiful forms. We are the soil waiting to be watered, so that we can erupt into a productive life.

I think of the potter at the wheel as a metaphor for the way in which we can form ourselves into any shape we like, once we have learned enough to know the options. Water as Knowledge brings forth the ability of Earth as Self to be a vessel of growth and change. Keep learning. Stay curious. Always wonder, and remember that all knowledge has value.

*Related entry:* *Haiku #21*

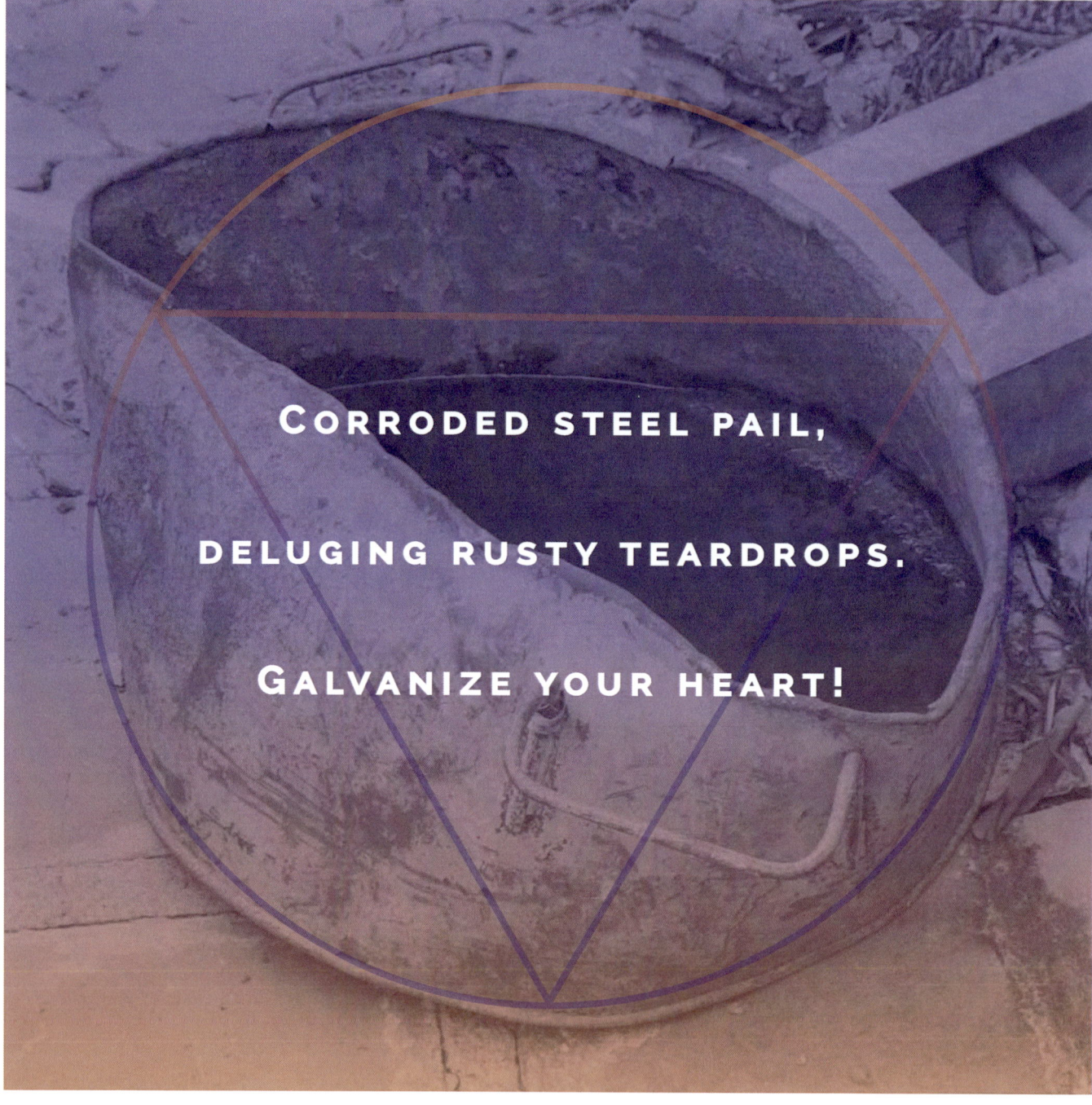

# #39 OF 49

## I PROFESS THAT — I SEE — INSPIRATION IN THE ACHIEVEMENTS OF OTHERS.

### AJÑA: WATER (I SEE) *TOUCHES* SVADISTHANA: METAL (I FEEL)

When Water impacts Metal it can have a corrosive effect: Rust. I understand this as jealousy, envy, discouragement, or frustration. In *Profession #33* I mentioned this would be coming up. I have struggled at times with seeing the success of others, especially if I perceive their situation as something undeserved. It's base, and I need to do better.

Remember that when you know something good about someone else that sparks negative feelings in yourself, you are hurting yourself, not them. It betrays a lack of gratitude for your own gifts. Rather than fill your bucket with sadness or contempt, consider how what you know about a person's happy situation can actually make you feel motivated to continue striving.

Galvanization has three definitions: Applying an electrifying motivation to spur someone emotionally into action; applying an electrical shock to the body to improve a medical condition (i.e., heart attacks, psychological/emotional problems, etc.); or to apply an electrical charge in order to plate iron or steel with a protective coating of zinc.

*Related entry:* **Haiku #41**

Scalding mists propel:

Burning thoughts revolve. Evolve!

Glistening pyre.

# #40 OF 49

## I PROFESS THAT — I SEE — THE IMPORTANCE OF CONSTANTLY REFINING MYSELF.

### AJÑA: WATER (I SEE) TOUCHES MANIPURA: FIRE (I DO)

I have an unhelpful habit wherein I think myself into torpor. I examine something so much that I become paralyzed. If your Water smothers your Fire, then all your wisdom and experience are for naught.

Rather than make this a negative exhortation not to do something (e.g., "don't extinguish your campfire"), I am going to consider another way water and heat can interact productively: Steam engines. Apply what you know, so that a perpetual cycle of learning and doing becomes an ever expanding practice of refinement. This constantly revolving cycle is what made me think of nuclear powered steam turbines that become more and more efficient as we learn to glean more and more power from them.

Notice that the words on each line specifically combine Water with Fire (scald = fire, mist = water, propel = fire; burn = fire, thought = water, revolve/evolve = fire; glisten = water, pyre = fire). It was important to me to emphasize how water does not drown fire; instead, both exist together to make more from each other synergistically.

*Related entry:* **Haiku #41**

Fishers casting nets:

Gathering, grasping joined thoughts.

Boats. Ripples. Shifts.

# #41 OF 49

## I PROFESS THAT — I SEE — COLLABORATION AS A PRACTICE RICH WITH POTENTIAL.

### AJÑA: WATER (I SEE) TOUCHES ANAHATA: WOOD (I LOVE)

When Water contacted Wood, my first impression was rot. I seem to have an initially negative connection with Water (ironic since I'm a Cancer, and that is Water's cardinal sign). My immediate impressions were rust in **#39**, extinguishment in **#40**, and now this? I guess I need to meditate on my relationship with knowledge and learning, which rather surprises me. Am I too rigid in my thinking? Probably.

Water with Wood conjures boats and other means of cooperative transportation. What are you shipping from your mind to the world? Where will you cruise? What realizations come from the collaborative brainstorming process, from rowing together toward a destination, or casting collective nets? How do these ripples force a shift in balance or perspective, revealing innovative solutions? Note that **#23** is also about collaboration. Profession #41 gathers ideas together, and **#23** describes the phase where those ideas are discussed and developed.

Note multiple entendres on "grasping" (holding/understanding), "joined" (paired/shared/enlisted), and "shifts" (taking turns to work/redirect/rebalance/change).

Saturated air

exudes dew. Humid musings:

Cling… Bead… Distend… Drip!

# #42 OF 49

## I PROFESS THAT — I SEE — MY KNOWLEDGE AND IDEAS AS VALUABLE GIFTS TO SHARE.

### AJÑA: WATER (I SEE) TOUCHES VISHUDHA: AIR (I SAY)

Compare this haiku with its inverse, Profession #30. Teaching and discussing are practically the same. I was a high school teacher and college professor, and my students taught me as least as much as I taught them.

Dew occurs when water fills air, reaching a saturation point: That moment where water has nowhere to go but out. That is why the image I see in my mind is teaching: You burst with knowledge that you want to share or help others discover. What gratified me most? Watching students soak up information and then find ways to use it. Back and forth we would talk, explain, ask, and answer.

You know so much cool stuff — you do. Please remember you are probably smarter than you give yourself credit for, and that you have so much wisdom to share. Help others dissipate mist, fog, and haze.

Oo! Notice all those "oo" vowels on the second line? "Oo!" is the expression I tend to say when I realize something delightful.

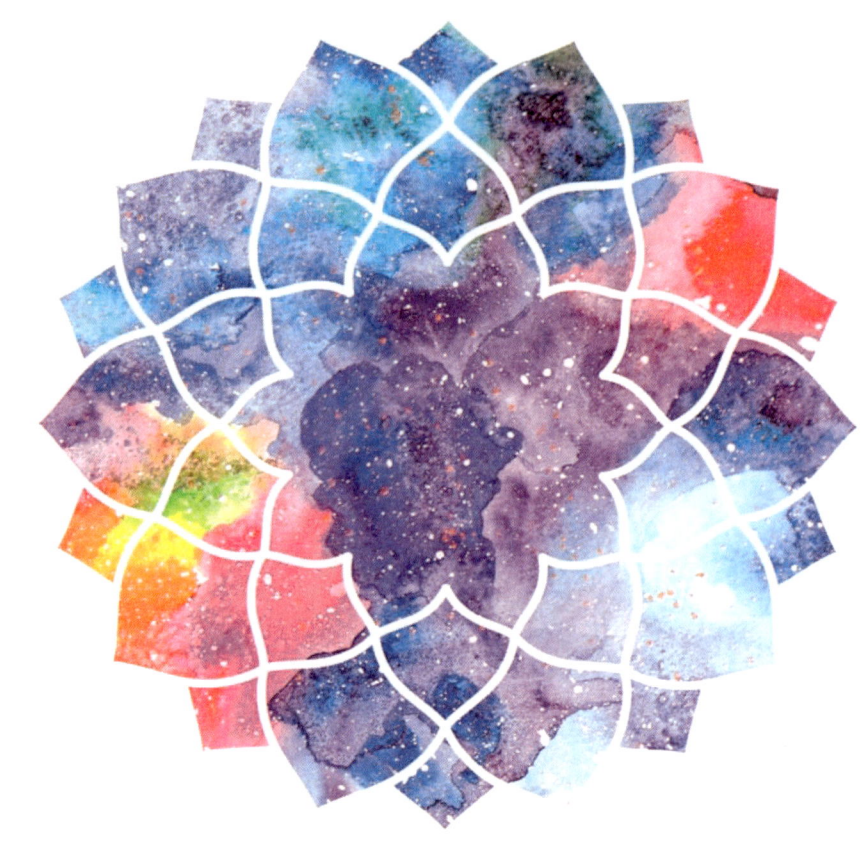

**COLOR**
PURPLE

**ELEMENTAL**
AKASHA

**PURPOSE**
ACCEPTING

**MANTRA**
"I KNOW"

# SAHASRARA
*Intro*

Also called the Crown Chakra, this energy vortex is located at the top of your scalp. Something interesting here is the difference between the Ajña manifestation of literal knowing and the Sahasrara manifestation of "I KNOW." Consider the difference between knowing in the mind versus knowing through the soul: I know that one day I will die, but I KNOW that it won't be the end of my journey. The distinction is between knowing and accepting, or between seeing and believing. Once you accept something, you take it as a matter of fact from a position of faith. I SEE/I know the universe is infinite. Also, I KNOW/I believe the universe is infinite. When your Crown Chakra is healthy and aligned you will profess serenely. Realization, acceptance, teaching, and guidance channel your spirit out into the wider sense of Being.

When it is misaligned you block your true Self with foolishness, rejection, secretiveness, and selfishness. But is there too much energy causing you to supernova, or not enough energy causing you to collapse into a black hole?

The seventh cycle of *The 49 Professions of Joy* redefines how you manifest your ideals. Are you fulfilling your sense of morality? Have you considered your purpose?

Whereas with Ajña the focus is on gaining information and learning, Sahasrara shares by teaching and guiding. Balance here bequeaths wisdom absorbed during experience. Whereas Muladhara grounds you firmly in the physical, that secure base allows Sahasrara to draw you gracefully toward the divine.

Galaxies collide,

never touch. I am. Am I?

Zero holds googol.

# #43 OF 49

## I PROFESS THAT — I KNOW — DYNAMIC BALANCE IS MORE IDEAL THAN STATIC PERFECTION.

*SAHASRARA: AKASHA (I KNOW) TOUCHES SAHASRARA: AKASHA (I KNOW)*

When Heaven touches Heaven all the forces of eternity mesh. When two galaxies "collide," from the outside it looks like they violently obliterate each other. However, there is such vast space between everything, anyone inside those galaxies would have almost no chance of knowing it. Two stars meeting would practically never happen. The time scale and physical distances are so vast and incomprehensible that one of the largest events possible in the universe would barely register, if at all.

Our entire solar system would be totally unchanged when Andromeda hits the Milky Way (assuming the Sun hasn't already eaten everything). That enormously dynamic nothing is like Nirvana. It is replete with paradoxes wherein all and none are combined to become the nothing that is: Zeroes that are the place holders of googolplex. Vibrating stillness, omniscient ignorance, dynamic torpor, apathetic bliss . . .

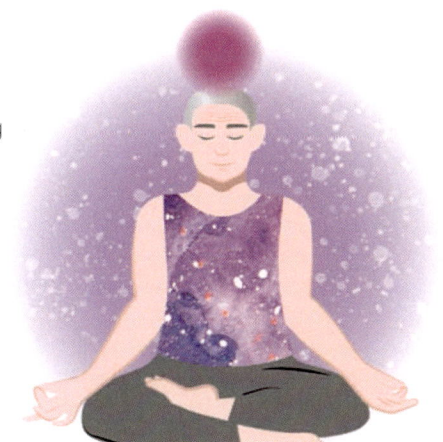

Muladhara states I AM. Sahasrara asks AM I? Ideal (according to dictionary.com): "A standard taken as a model for imitation that exists only in the imagination."

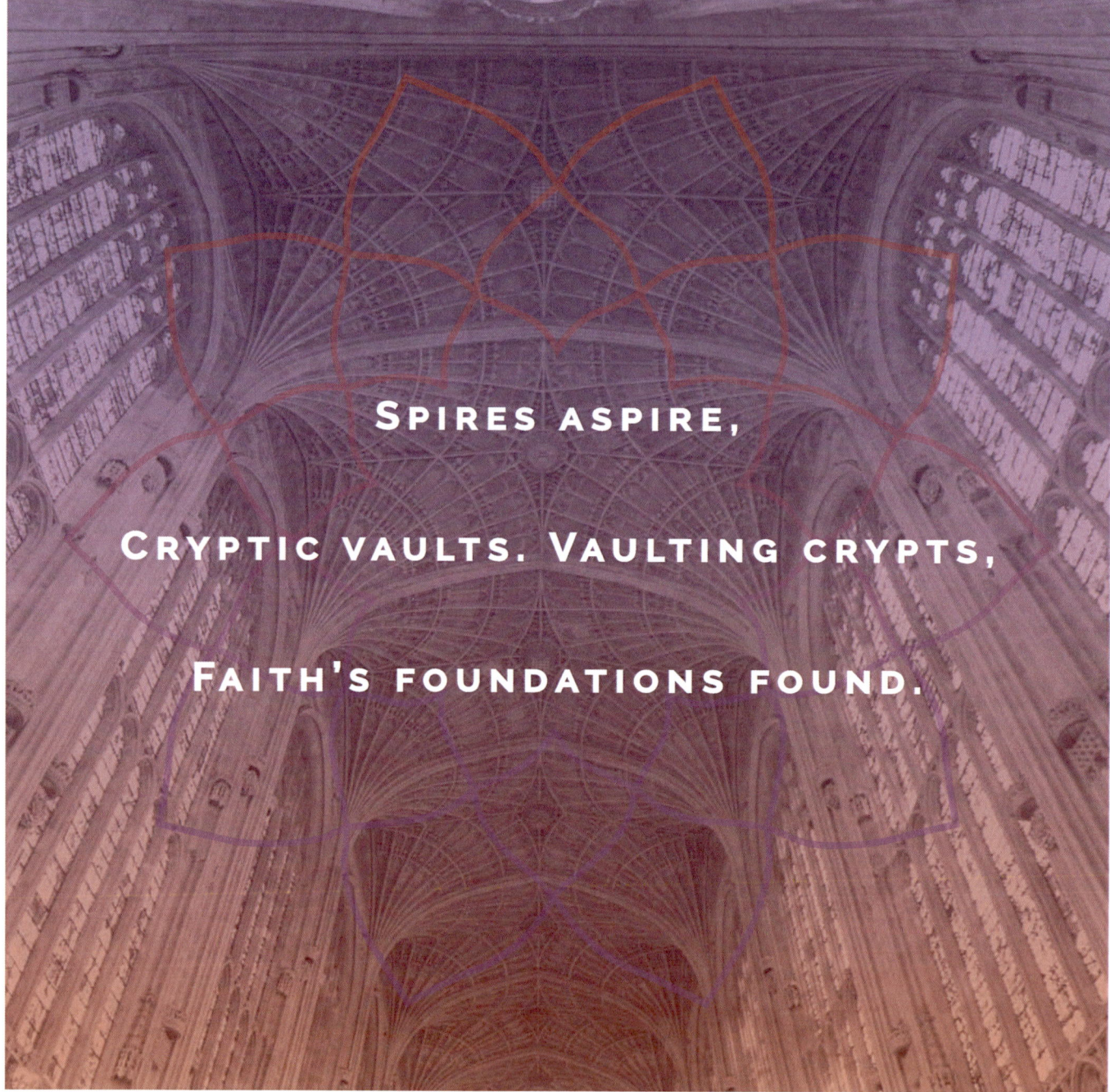

# #44 OF 49

## I PROFESS THAT — I KNOW — THAT I DESERVE RESPECT AS I ASPIRE TO FULFILL MY POTENTIAL.

### SAHASRARA: AKASHA (I KNOW) TOUCHES MULADHARA: EARTH (I AM)

When Sahasrara influences Muladhara, the eternal/divine directs itself toward our sense of self, well-being, and health. A popular notion: Your body itself is a temple. Treat it with respect and reverence.

In cathedrals we experience the formless divine inside a space enclosed by formed rock. That is a manifestation of the idea that God is present in Earth itself: "Aspire" contains spire. We are the sacred spaces, so rock is also enclosed in divinity.

Our spirits deserve love, care, and praise. Our bodies merit adoration, awe, and wonder. As in **Profession #7**, we ourselves are in simultaneous contact with the profane and the divine. In that haiku we conceive of and exist in both realms, but in this haiku we are the actual stuff of these places. Remember **Profession #1** as well.

Stone forms the physical tower literally building toward heaven, but spiritual yearning is what conceptually anchors the deepest core of belief. Both your body and your spirit seek trustworthy stability. "Foundation" contains found.

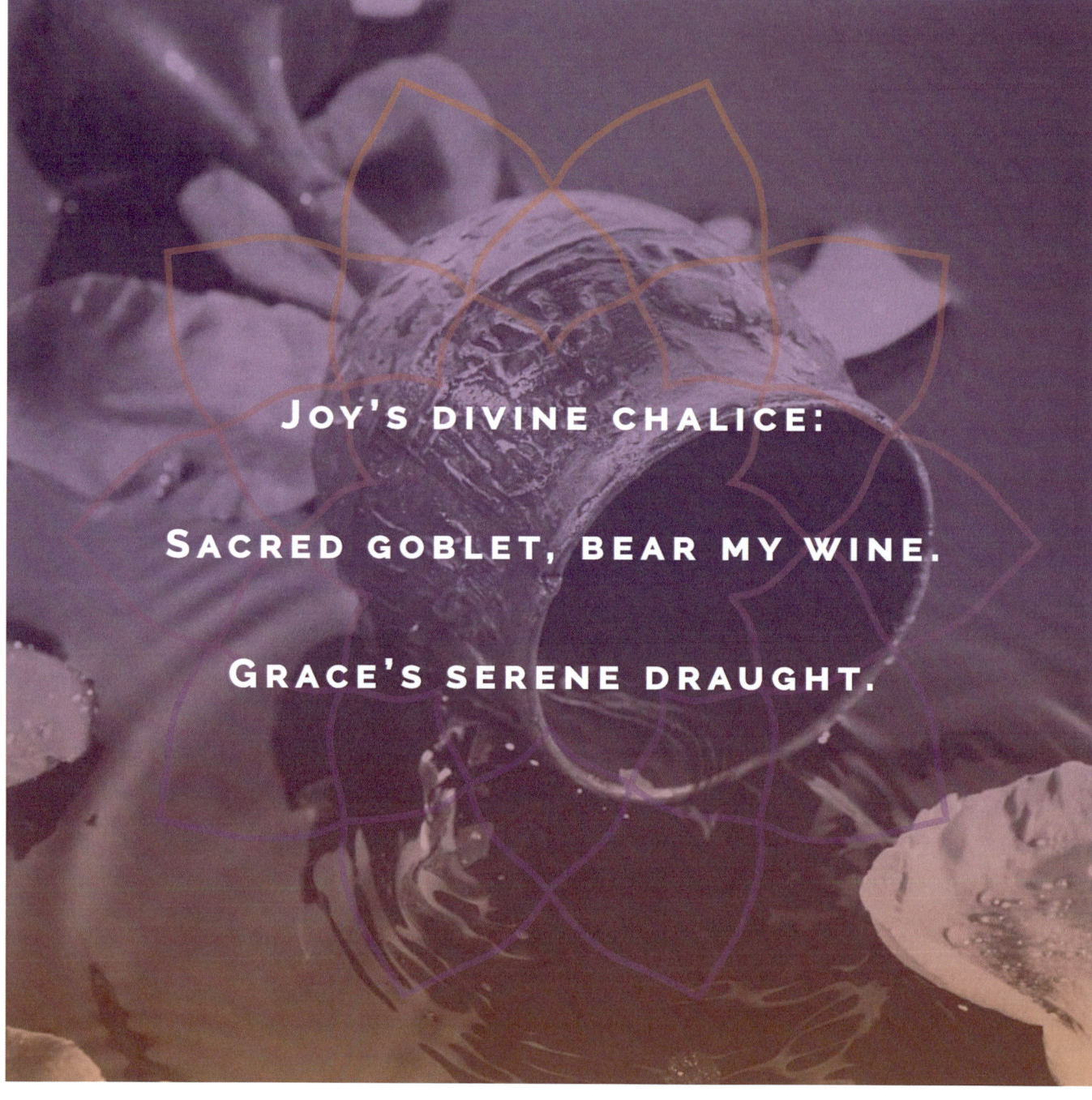

# #45 OF 49

## I PROFESS THAT — I KNOW — MY FEELINGS ARE AN HONEST EXPRESSION OF MYSELF.

### SAHASRARA: AKASHA (I KNOW) TOUCHES SVADISTHANA: METAL (I FEEL)

When Akasha imbues Metal, sacred objects are forged. What is sacred here? Pleasure, joy, and intuition. When faithfully imbibed as they are, they create relieved contentment.

The self acceptance pouring from our sacramental chalices reinforces our trust in ourselves. Feeling that our feelings are healthy is intoxicating, especially if you have not allowed yourself that pleasure. When I have drunk this nectar deeply, it fills my belly with gratitude like a soothing elixir. Remember to gulp your fill of this liquid confidence, especially when it isn't easy.

When I feel I cannot trust myself or my choices, despite them being logically sound, I look at my cat. What is she doing? She's sleeping on the couch usually. What does that mean? Nothing is wrong. I have a safe home, I am not hungry, ISIS isn't busting through the door with bombs and crazed hatred. Whatever seems so dire to me cannot be that bad or else kitty would be fretting. She is a good barometer of reality.

Sharp, beckoning guide:

Your flame's blade lacerates gloom,

parries knife-edged rocks.

# #46 OF 49

## I PROFESS THAT — I KNOW — MY ACTIONS MOTIVATE OTHERS TO PERFORM GOODNESS.

### SAHASRARA: AKASHA (I KNOW) TOUCHES MANIPURA: FIRE (I DO)

In *Profession #34* I asked you to express ideas that inspire others to acts of kindness. In this poem your actions, not your words, set the example. Here we look at how morality affects choice. That is to say, how do your beliefs and sense of connection to the universe affect what you do?

In *Profession #19*, the question was how do you act upon your beliefs. That isn't the same. They are very closely related, but this haiku is a change in direction. As opposed to cautioning you against zealotry, here I am encouraging you to be the beacon in the dark. Do what you know to be right, even in the face of adversity.

Let your moral code be the guiding light in your own life, and hopefully an influence upon others who may be floundering. Depression, loneliness, callousness, greed, cruelty: Those are dangerous waters to navigate. Be the stedfast lighthouse seeking to help others avoid crashing on their internal crags. Shine a lighter example.

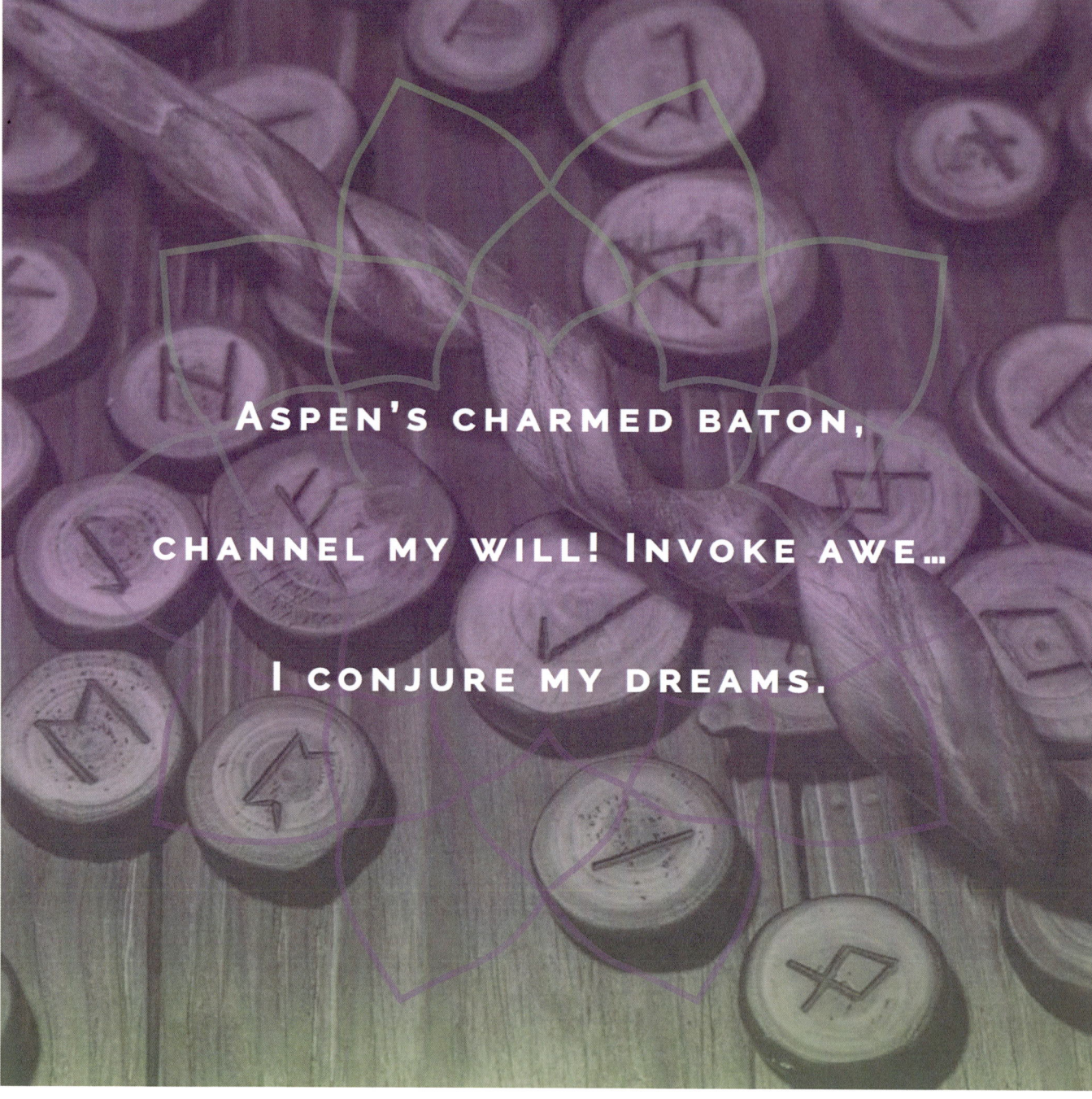

Aspen's charmed baton, channel my will! Invoke awe... I conjure my dreams.

# #47 OF 49

## I PROFESS THAT — I KNOW — I AM CONNECTED TO THE WORLD AND EVERYONE IN IT.

**SAHASRARA: AKASHA (I KNOW)** TOUCHES **ANAHATA: WOOD (I LOVE)**

The ethereal element's influence on wood: Wands. They are a powerful tool for focusing intention. You yourself are the conduit, but props are fun!

Whether or not the metaphysical practice of Attraction appeals to you, it is quite plain that defining what you want, bringing your various resources to bear on it, and keeping a clear focus on it is what gives your goals a chance at life. But you must actively create your opportunities. Be the lightning rod of success! How will you share that bounty? Imagining how your eventual largesse can improve the world is a fantastic motivator.

If it helps you to use beads, runes, wands, or staves, then use them. Whatever object or activity helps you focus your inherent creativity, imbue it from your deep well of manifestation. Wands and other props serve as a useful reminder that you are connected to and part of the intentions that comprise every fiber of your body and every impulse in your mind.

Atmospheric chants

intone diaphanous prayers.

Dancing, colored hymns.

# #48 OF 49

## I PROFESS THAT — I KNOW — MY VOICE MATTERS, AND THAT IT CAN HELP OTHERS.

### SAHASRARA: AKASHA (I KNOW) TOUCHES VISHUDHA: AIR (I SAY)

When Sahasrara touches Vishudha, philosophical conversations, prayers, and sacred music give voice to what we want to express about our connection to eternity. I also was thinking about how heaven literally touches air when solar winds interact with our atmosphere.

The aurora borealis is a result of universal forces (electromagnetism) exciting colorful reactions over polar skies. They are a visible manifestation of our atmosphere protecting us from various universal powers. In my manner of thinking, it seemed like a nice image to conflate the northern lights with Gregorian chants.

These chants often focus on pleadings for mercy, protection, and salvation, so why not play with the double entendre in "atmospheric?" Why not imagine what our prayers might look or sound like to whichever gods might be watching or listening?

I am a very transparent person. I share to a fault. But I deeply value honesty, even when being truthful is embarrassing, controversial, or inconvenient. I would be remiss not to mention honesty as a mixing of Akasha and Air.

Ozone. Thunder... hush.

Electric tension... listen.

Cascading rain... learn.

# #49 OF 49

## I PROFESS THAT — I KNOW — MY STRENGTHS AND WEAKNESSES TEACH ME ABOUT MY WEAKNESSES AND STRENGTHS.

*SAHASRARA: AKASHA (I KNOW)* TOUCHES *AJÑA: WATER (I SEE)*

Whether it be delicate patters of small insights or a deluge of realization, we should constantly learn about ourselves. Collect all the droplets you can. Your puddles become pools, ponds, and lakes. Perhaps oceans one day?

Some valuable practices to gain insight into yourself include meditation, therapy, reading a wide variety of materials, and working with life or career coaches. I have been very lucky in recent years to have found a therapist who is helpful and compatible. I cannot stress enough how important it is to know yourself honestly.

Self actualization helps with healing wounds, growing personally, and refining perspective. I liken it to the onset of a summer shower. Realizing something is amiss in myself — like the calm before a rain. I need to quiet myself to sense whatever comes. Then there's the tension, knowing I am about to see or think something that could be transformative. And then finally rain bursts, and I get drenched in new information.

I wish you lifelong introspection.

# ABOUT *Haiku*

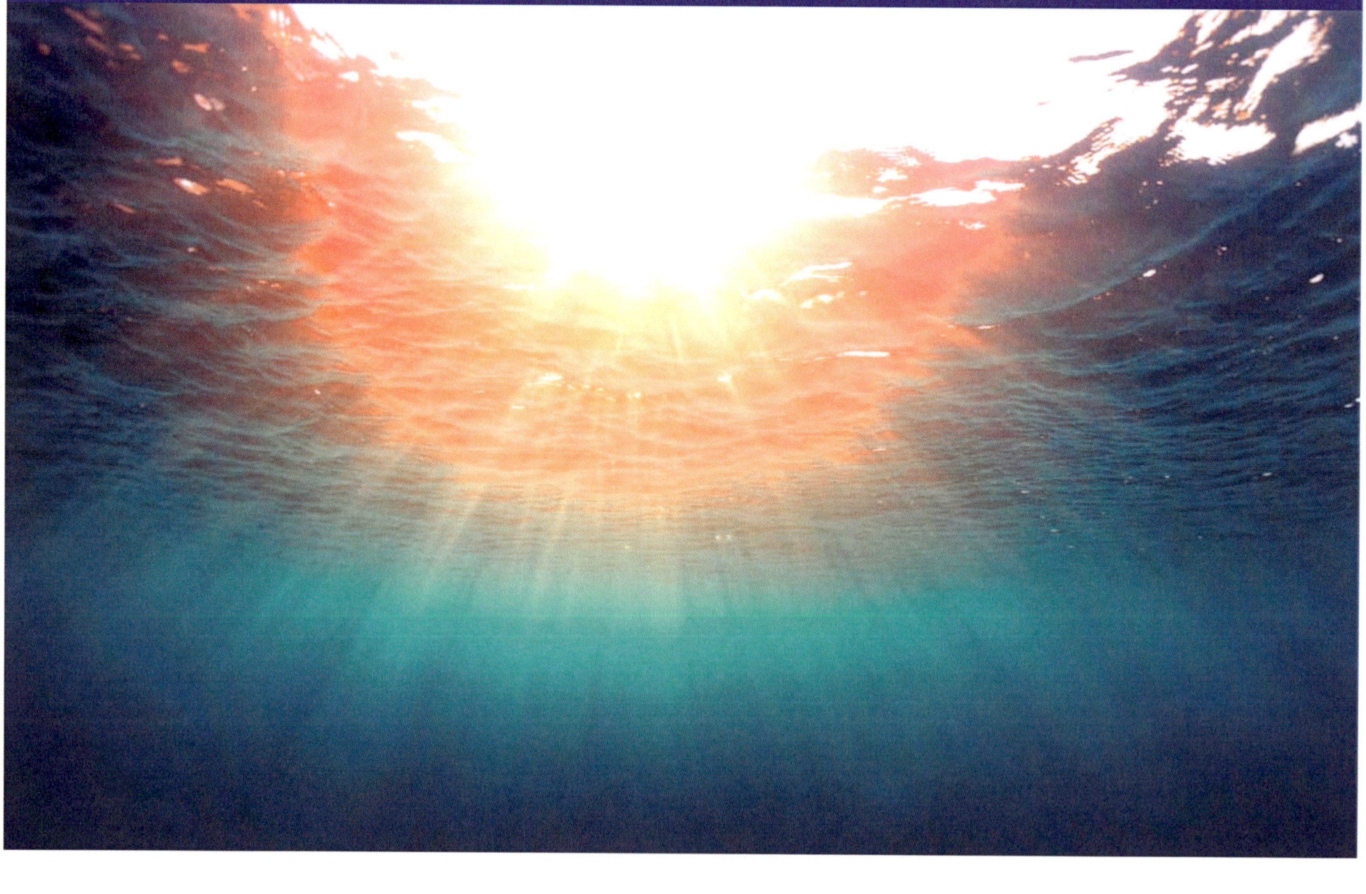

A salient feature of traditional Japanese aesthetic is a focus on the essential. Removing all superfluous, distracting detail. The technique and discipline of diminution, not accumulation.

Haiku is a classical Japanese poetry form going back centuries. But beyond the superficial structure, there exists a distinct commitment to saying as much as possible with as few words as possible. I do not speak Japanese at all, so there is a great deal of etiquette that proves impossible for me. For example, depending on the season of the year when you write your poem, certain syllables on particular lines are required. I cannot use katakana or hiragana, so that expectation is futile in my work. In its place, I impose stylistic boundaries on myself.

**Structure**: Haiku are generally thought of as having three lines. The first line has five syllables. The second has seven, and the last also has five. This gives a total of 17 syllables.

**Imagery**: Most of the haiku I have read take images from the natural world. Whether it be plants, animals, insects, geographic features, seasons, clouds, or weather, many poems look at the ambient environment for source material. Also, there are plenty that look at circumstances, behaviors, buildings, and picturesque scenes.

**Metaphors**: Whatever the imagery, haiku often take that external information and translate it or emphasize it in such a way that it becomes an artful observation about philosophy. They are succinct descriptions of truth, irony, spirituality, humanity, or culture delivered by way of a "simple" evocation.

# ADVICE FOR Writing Your Own

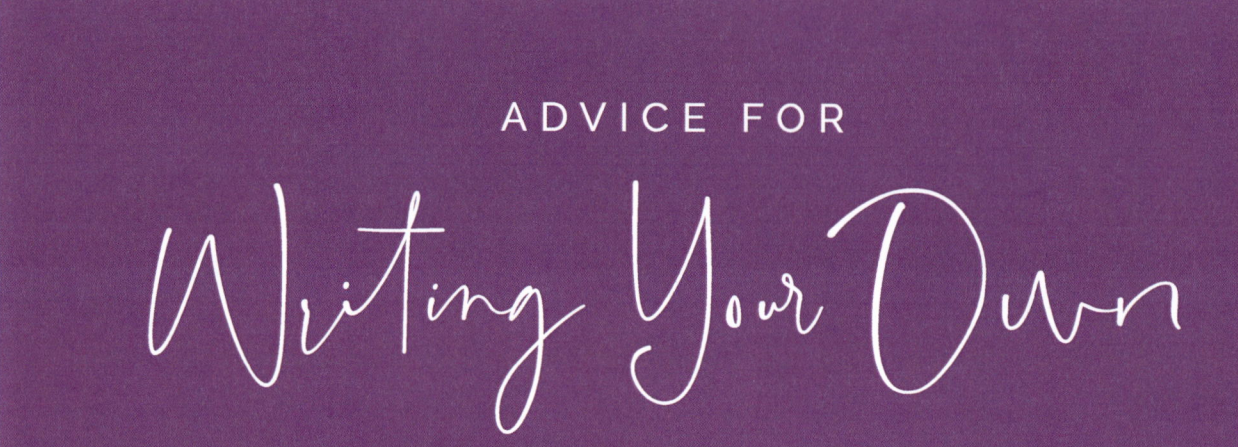

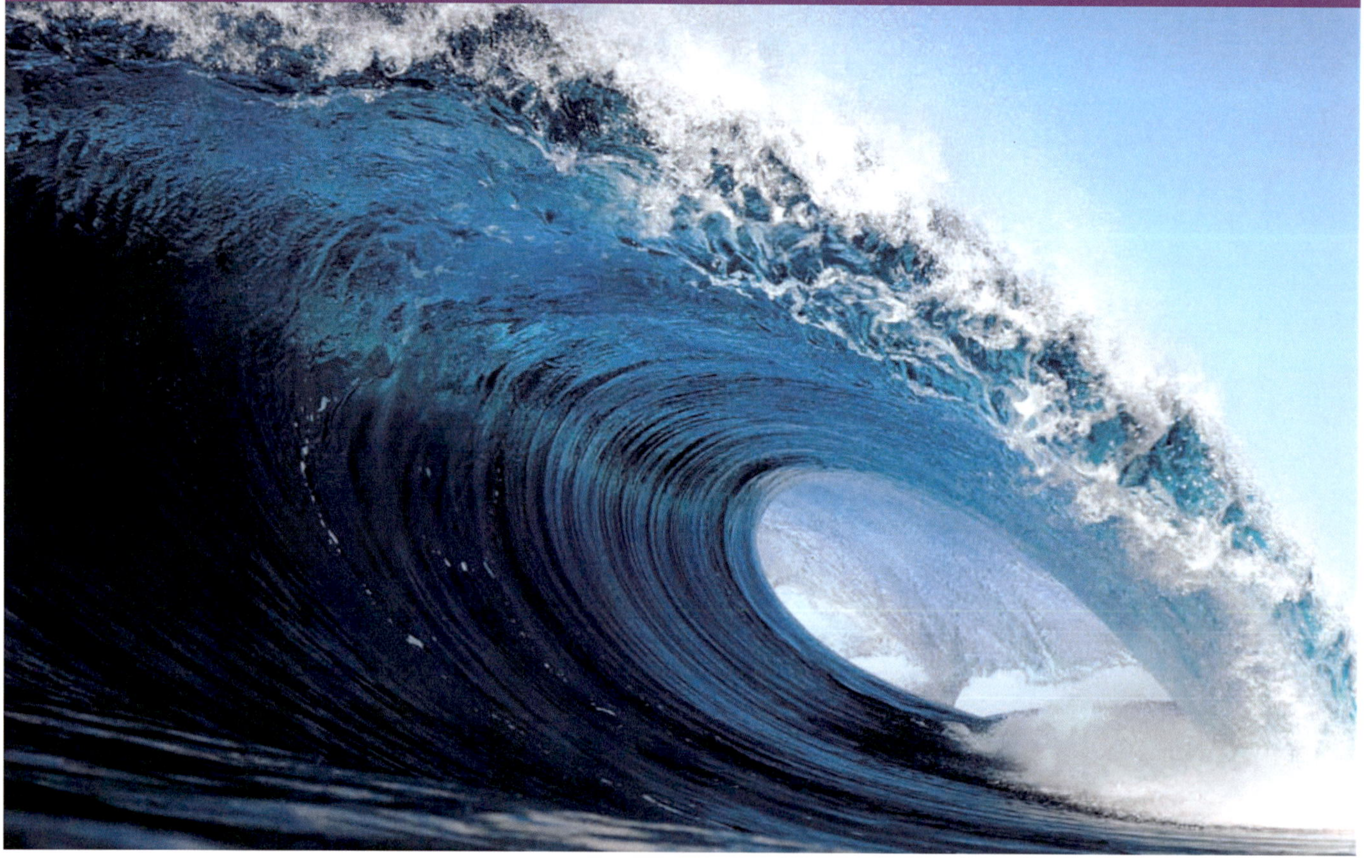

There are no rules to enjoying creative writing. However, if you aspire toward something more studied, it helps to rein in the billions of possibilities. Cute though they are, you gotta herd as few kittens as possible!

It was grueling to write these haiku, because I exercised discipline to develop my style — my OCD chakra is *definitely* aligned now. I say "grueling" with affection: It was extremely rewarding and gratifying. If I haven't terrified you off writing your own, please share them to the *Facebook Page: The 49 Professions of Joy*.

**Economy of Language**: You have 17 syllables to accomplish many tasks simultaneously. You have to create a scene, conjure a mood, work within coherent themes, and make a broader point artfully. Although intimidating, it makes the investment even more valuable.

**Wasted Syllables**: You have no wiggle room. Abandon all extraneous syllables. Focus on nouns, verbs, adjectives, and adverbs. Exclude articles (a/an/the), prepositions (to/from/by/in/on/under/beyond/etc.), conjunctions (so/but/and/because/etc.), demonstrative adjectives (this/those/etc.), pronouns (we/it/them/etc.), auxiliary verbs (be/have/can/will/might/etc.), and infinitives (to go/to see/etc.).

Compare two examples of five syllables: 1) I am happy now; 2) Happily gazing. The first is full of redundancies and wasted syllables. It offers no depth or nuance. The second assumes "I am," provides "now," and leaves room to begin telling a story by including action. The first: Dead stop. The second provides options, entrances.

www.ingramcontent.com/pod-product-compliance
Lightning Source LLC
Chambersburg PA
CBRC090746010526
44114CB00008B/98